THE 17 DAY DIET

A DOCTOR'S PLAN DESIGNED TO TARGET
BOTH BELLY FAT AND VISCERAL FAT
FOR FAST RESULTS THAT LAST!

DR. MIKE MORENO

RODALE.

Exclusive direct mail edition published by Rodale Inc. in 2012 in arrangement with Free Press, a division of Simon & Schuster, Inc.
© 2010, 2012 by 17 Day Diet, Inc.

Library of Congress Cataloging-in-Publication Data is on file with the publisher.
ISBN-13: 978–1–60961–916–9

2 4 6 8 10 9 7 5 3   hardcover

We inspire and enable people to improve their lives and the world around them.
rodalebooks.com

I dedicate this book to my family and friends who have supported me and my dreams, but most important to my mother and father who always encouraged and supported me. They placed a big emphasis on education, and instilled in me the importance of hard work and helping others. I would also like to thank my patients for providing me with the motivation to think outside the box, in hopes of making this world a healthier happier place.

Contents

• • • • • • • • • •

PART III Make It Stick

Acknowledgments

• •

I feel a deep sense of gratitude to Maggie Greenwood-Robinson. Without her persistence and endless hours of dedication to this project, the book you are holding in your hands may not have been written. I'd also like to thank the many people involved in putting the program and its support materials together.

My hope is that this book will help make the world a healthier and happier place. It's never too late to be fit and fabulous!

PART I

....

The 17 Day Diet

1

Just Give Me 17 Days

I can personally sum up the 17 Day Diet in two words: fast results. Depending on your weight when you start out and your metabolism, you might expect to lose up to 10 to 12 pounds the first 17 days. Of course, the further you are from your ideal weight, the more you'll lose initially.

Let's not kid each other: When you start a diet, you want to see results right away, in how you look and in how you feel. That's because our society is geared toward the immediate; we want things and we want them now. The same is true of weight loss. We get impatient when the pounds don't come off fast enough to meet our expectations. It seems much easier to give up than to go on.

This diet is designed to produce quick results, not because it starves you down to size but because its carefully designed balance of food and exercise adjusts your body metabolically so that you burn fat, day in and day out.

Also important: The weight-reduction portion of this diet is limited to just 17 days at a time so that you aren't demoralized by the thought of endless months of dieting.

Nor are you apt to plateau like you often do on other diets. The 17 Day Diet keeps your body and metabolism guessing. I call this "body confusion." With each 17 Day Cycle, you're changing your calorie count and the foods you eat. By varying these things, you prevent your body from adapting. The scale is less likely to get stuck. The added bonus: You'll never get bored. And it's fun watching those pounds melt off. So confusion is good!

At the end of 17 days, you'll go on to a second 17 Day Cycle, then a third, and finally enter the weight-stabilization Cycle of the diet in which you get to eat a greater variety of foods, including your favorite foods *within reason.* (I don't want you to get too chummy with the all-you-can-eat buffets again.)

I already know what you're thinking: Is it possible to shed pounds swiftly yet safely? If done right, without sacrificing good nutrition, the answer is yes.

Despite what many nutritionists have preached for years, rapid weight-loss diets can be healthy if done correctly and can work wonders on reducing pounds and inches in just days. Brand-new research

MISTER MD, CAN YOU PLEASE TELL ME ?

But won't a lot of the weight I lose be water weight?

Yes! And that's awesome, because water is weight too. Never dismiss those extra pounds as only "water weight"; this is a self-defeating attitude. Cosmetically, water weight can hide fat loss and be particularly frustrating. Healthwise, fluid retention can put a strain on your heart. When your body holds water, this means there's more water in your blood. Your heart has to work harder to pump all that extra volume. Once all that excess fluid has disappeared, so will your bloat and puffiness. You'll start looking visibly thinner in three or four days. And chances are, you'll feel much lighter and be more motivated to watch what you eat.

suggests that the faster you take weight off, the longer you keep it off. Now that's a reason for dieters everywhere to rejoice. Plus, if you're too embarrassed by a recent weight spike or have just gained an embarrassing eight pounds after a holiday weekend or an ice cream binge, this diet can get you back on track fast.

The 17 Day Diet thus gives your body the perfect jump-start, the

SCIENCE SAYS: Slow Isn't Necessarily Better

Conventional wisdom says that rapid weight loss leads to rapid weight regain. A new generation of science, however, shows that slow isn't necessarily better.

Shape Up the Fast Way. A 2010 study from the University of Florida suggests that the key to long-term weight loss and maintenance is to lose weight quickly, not gradually. Among 262 obese middle-aged women, fast weight losers were those who shed more than 2 pounds a week. Compared to more gradual losers, fast weight losers lost more weight overall, maintained their weight loss longer and were less likely to put weight back on. The findings were published in the *International Journal of Behavioral Medicine*.

Trim Belly Fat. We pack on two forms of belly fat. One type collects around internal organs (also known as visceral fat). This type of fat raises blood pressure and cholesterol levels, and increases the risk of diabetes, Alzheimer's and even some cancers. Visceral fat is far more sinister than fat elsewhere in the body.

The other type sits just under the skin and is known as subcutaneous abdominal fat. It causes a hard-to-get-rid-of belly pouch. In a Finnish study published in the *International Journal of Obesity and Related Metabolic Disorders*, a rapid weight-loss diet followed for 6 weeks trimmed visceral abdominal fat by 25 percent and subcutaneous abdominal fat by 16 percent.

kind of quick drop in weight that gives you a powerful mental boost. My whole focus is to get you thin as soon as I can. When I do, just think: You'll no longer have to move around hauling the equivalent of two 40-pound bags of cement on your body. The button of your jeans will no longer pop out and ping off the wall. You'll no longer have to wear plus-sized clothing with those expandable waistlines. This diet will make you slim, healthy and curvy, and I won't make you slurp your way to a thinner you, or follow some hardcore exercise regime used by the Navy SEALs.

But you do have to accept that this won't be a pleasure diet. You've got to stop eating unhealthy crap. You've got to eat vegetables, fruit and lean meat. I'm not going to ask you to probe your inner eater and uncover hidden emotional reasons for why you're fat. But I am going to ask you to keep your portions down, cut your intake of fatty, sugary, salty foods and move your butt. You won't be faint with hunger or found in the kitchen at midnight, feeding on Froot Loops and tubes of cookie dough. You can do this, because anyone can do anything for 17 days.

The beauty of this program is that you won't get discouraged or bored by the prospect of staying on a diet for what seems like forever. It can yield results that will stand the test of time just as well as those long-term diets that emphasize depressingly slow incremental drops in weight. You'll love the fact that in 7, 10 or 17 days, you'll be slimmer. And chances are, you'll feel a lot lighter and have an absurd amount of energy.

The 17 Day Diet is doable and easy—unlike so many other diets, which are slightly less complicated than the checklist for a shuttle launch.

So can you just give me 17 days?

If you can, congratulations! You won't be disappointed.

What Lies Ahead?

So what is this 17 Day Diet? I'll go into depth in the next few chapters, but as a very quick summary, the 17 Day Diet is a fun, fantastic way of eating designed to take off weight quickly. It's based on some very simple principles, one of which is eating foods that favor fat-burning and are friendly to your digestive system.

I want to emphasize that excess weight is always a sign of nutritional and metabolic imbalance. Contrary to popular assumption, it's not strictly a question of how much exercise you do or how much food you eat. Rather, it's also a question of what types of foods are eaten, and how they are digested, assimilated and metabolized. If any of these components of good nutrition are compromised, then the body will not be adequately nourished at the cellular level, metabolic function will be impaired and toxins will accumulate. Thus, to lose weight fast we need to optimize digestion and metabolism. That's what the 17 Day Diet does.

Trust me, you'll love the rapid loss of a few pounds so much that you'll decide to keep on going. After the first 17 days, there's another 17 days, and another—3 total Cycles and a maintenance Cycle in which you get to eat whatever the heck you want, mainly on weekends. Here's an overview:

Quick and Easy Overview of the 17 Day Diet	
Cycles	Purpose
Cycle 1: Accelerate (17 days)	To promote rapid weight loss by improving digestive health. It helps clear sugar from the blood to boost fat-burning and discourage fat storage.
Cycle 2: Activate (17 days)	To reset your metabolism through a strategy that involves increasing and decreasing your caloric consumption to stimulate fat-burning and to help prevent plateaus.
Cycle 3: Achieve (17 days)	To develop good eating habits through the re-introduction of additional foods and move you closer to your goal weight.
Cycle 4: Arrive (ongoing)	To keep you at your goal weight through a program of eating that lets you enjoy your favorite foods on weekends, while eating healthfully during the week.

Once we're through with all the basics, I'm going to talk to you about how to follow the diet. I can't wait to show you all of its wonderful components and start you on your way to looking fit and fabulous. Take it one step at a time so that you don't get overwhelmed.

Your Appointment with Me

I might as well take a moment here to introduce myself. I'm a family practice doctor. Under America's health insurance system, most people go first to a doctor like me for all complaints, from infections to chronic illnesses. I love the diversity of family practice. One moment, I'm treating an 18-year-old guy with the flu; the next, a 90-year-old woman with joint pain.

I became a doctor for the reasons most people do—because I wanted to save lives, pure and simple. In my heart of hearts, I believe a doctor is so much more than a person who dispenses medication or marks off symptoms like a checklist at a sushi bar. He or she should treat the whole person. I make it a point to get to know each patient as a person before I put a stethoscope to his or her chest.

I run my office a little differently than most places. Nowadays, you spend more time waiting in the examining room than you did in the waiting room. In fact, you spend more time in the examining room than the person who decorated it. It's almost like going to a restaurant and being told that, even though you have a reservation, you have to sit at the bar for a while. The only difference is that in the doctor's office, no one offers you a cocktail, and you have to wear a boxy blue paper exam gown that opens in the front.

The next time you have to wait in the examining room, do some fun things to pass the time. Glue the tongue depressors together into coasters and sell them to other patients. Or peel off all the wallpaper without disturbing any of the diplomas.

I do things differently in my office. My patients don't wait forever.

My patients oftentimes don't even sit on the examining table when I talk to them. I sit on the examining table and they get the comfortable chair. The butcher paper upholstering the examining table is wonderful to draw on. Sometimes I hop off the table and start drawing pictures of organs to explain things to patients.

I'm responsible for 2,000 patients, though not all in one day. Many of them are women, and 80 percent of my new patients are overweight. Most know it. One of the things I've always found interesting is that my patients often come in with a complaint of back pain, or knee pain or just plain old fatigue. Before I can get a word out, they say, "I know it's because I'm fat." Patients are smart.

Ever since I became a doctor, I've always been concerned with prevention. Prevention is the doorway to longevity. I hate shoving medications at problems that can be fixed with simple changes in lifestyle.

A good example is a patient I'll call Sharon, age 60. Sharon has type 2 diabetes. When I first started seeing her, she was taking oral diabetes medication. Once she changed to a healthier diet and started walking regularly with a friend, she was able to get off all her meds. What a triumph that was!

Then about a year ago, Sharon came in for her regular appointment. We reviewed the results of her latest blood work. Her sugars were through the roof. Her A1C test, which reflects a patient's blood sugar over the past 90 days, was suddenly out of range.

What on earth had happened?

As we talked, Sharon told me that she no longer had a walking partner so she quit exercising altogether.

"I'll walk with you!" I volunteered. I couldn't bear to see her health slip. And so I became her walking partner. Before long, others joined us. Our walking group became affectionately known as *Walk with Your Doc* and has swelled to sometimes more than 50 people of all ages. We walk every Tuesday and Thursday morning without fail. I love it, because I thrive on helping people live full, healthy, active lives.

Of course, a huge part of prevention is weight management. You see, the death toll racked up by heart disease, high blood pressure, stroke, diabetes, and all the other fat-related diseases is scary. Studies even associate obesity with poor immune function. That makes overweight people more susceptible to infections and cancer. Obesity will kill far more Americans each year than any terrorist would dare dream of taking out.

Everybody knows this. I'm just bringing it up again to remind you that tubs of ice cream and bags full of chips are not worth shortening your life over.

We're already in so much trouble with trans fats, cheap sugars, excess sodium, and unpronounceable additives jazzing up junk food—stuff that causes your arteries to clog up like rusty pipes. With every-

MISTER MD, CAN YOU PLEASE TELL ME ?

Do I have to exercise while on the 17 Day Diet?

Yes, but I won't be asking you to sweat to golden oldies, pump it up or feel the burn. In other words—no overexercising. Since you'll be scaling back on calories, you should do less exercising, or else you'll get too run down and sore, especially during the first two Cycles. I will ask you, however, to do just 17 minutes a day of easy exercising like walking.

The 17 Day Diet has a companion exercise DVD called *The 17 Minute Workout* that you can purchase from our website, www.the17daydiet. com. It's cardio-based and geared toward pure fat-burning.

So put down this book. Do this workout, or go outside and walk around your neighborhood for 17 minutes. Then come back and pick up where you left off.

thing plaguing the American diet, I had to concentrate on creating a program that would be safe and effective, and produce quick but lasting results. People had to get the weight off, then learn how to keep it off. I didn't want to tell my patients to go on this diet or that diet because many diets out there are nutritionally unbalanced, are hard to follow or just don't work fast enough to keep you motivated.

Thus, the 17 Day Diet evolved. It uses the latest medical knowledge on nutrition, foods and what the body needs for successful weight loss and good health.

Let me add here: You should check with your own physician before starting this program. Your doctor knows what's best for you. Based on my experience with my own patients, most people who have gotten out of shape over the years can follow the 17 Day Diet and do very well on it, though results can vary.

There Is More to Love about the 17 Day Diet . . .

Whether you've got 10 pounds to lose or a hundred, being overweight is one of life's lesser joys. It affects every aspect of your life, maybe some things you never thought about. When you lose weight, practically everything in your life will change for the better. Let's talk about this now.

Get a Healthy Bod

You're going to be focused on losing pounds and inches. Some days, you might get a little discouraged if the scale doesn't move down fast enough, even though this diet does help prevent plateaus. But there's absolutely nothing to be discouraged about. There are other wonderful things happening inside your body that won't be reflected on the scale, like your blood pressure, blood sugar and cholesterol decreasing.

Okay, I realize that right now you might not care about these things. You just want to slip into that sexy black number hanging in your closet . . . you know, the one that used to fit years ago. But it's important to understand that your weight and health are not separate issues. Being overweight is a symptom of being unhealthy. Focus on your weight and your health will improve—instantly. Consider what the results of various research studies say about the rather immediate effects of healthy nutrition on the body:

After 15 minutes: After the first morning of eating a healthy breakfast, your stomach's satiety signals have registered in your brain, and you feel full. The body's internal chemistry is at its most active first thing in the morning, so your breakfast is then used to the maximum. If you eliminated processed foods (white bread, sugary cereals) for whole grains and lean proteins like egg whites, along with fresh fruit, you should feel energetic and mentally alert after just one meal.

After 3 hours: Your artery linings are able to expand sufficiently to increase blood flow to the body's tissues and organs.

After 6 hours: The HDL (happy cholesterol) in your blood perks up and starts scouring LDL (lousy cholesterol) from the blood. You can think of LDLs as delivery trucks, depositing cholesterol in blood vessels, and HDLs as garbage trucks, taking them back to the liver, where they're broken down.

After 12 hours: Your body finally has an opportunity to burn the fat it has stored for energy because you've eliminated sugar. When you're eating a lot of sugar, your body is so busy processing the sugar that it doesn't have time to do its other job, which is to help the body burn fat. So guess what? The fat ends up hanging around.

After 16 hours: You get a restful night's sleep.

After 24 hours: You're 1 to 2 pounds lighter, because your body has begun to flush excess water and toxins from your system.

After 3 days: Once your body senses it's losing weight, its blood-related numbers (cholesterol, blood pressure, blood sugar) start traveling in a healthy direction.

After 1 week: Your cholesterol levels can drop significantly. Blood levels of important disease-fighting antioxidants like vitamin C and vitamin E are higher. Your bowels are in better working order, and you should be at least 5 pounds lighter.

After 2 weeks: You'll experience healthy drops in blood pressure if you've been diagnosed with hypertension. Expect to have lost up to 10 pounds by now.

After 1 month: Nobody has to filter out chunks of fast food from your blood anymore. By now, blood levels of LDL cholesterol can fall by nearly 30 percent—a drop similar to that seen with some cholesterol-lowering drugs.

After 6 weeks: You've lost so much weight you can't buy new, smaller clothes fast enough. Yes, you should have lost quite a bit of weight (20 pounds is not unusual), and your blood cholesterol and triglyceride levels will be substantially improved.

After 12 weeks: Many significant health numbers—cholesterol, triglycerides (fat in the blood), blood pressure, glucose and insulin—should begin to, if not completely, normalize.

After 6 months: You'll feel healthier because your body will be retaining more vitamins and minerals. Because you reduced your sugar intake significantly over this period, insulin production will have normalized. So your risk of developing type 2 diabetes is reduced, as this can be linked to a larger intake of sugar. Your energy levels have improved dramatically because your body has

GET SKINNY SHORTCUT

Posture Stand up straight. Not only does slouching make your belly protrude, but it gives your core muscles an undeserved break. Standing erect, with the stomach held in, encourages the abs to work and can make you look slimmer naturally—and in an instant.

gone through a detoxing process. You've probably reached your goal. The hardest work is over, and now it's time to learn how to eat to maintain your newly slender silhouette.

Pretty amazing what a good diet can do, right? Don't you want all of this? Be brutally honest here: if you really want something you'll find a way to get it. So if you find yourself saying, "I didn't have time to prepare healthy food," let me ask you this: would you have found time if your life depended on it? Well, it does.

Get Sexy

When you're fit and in shape, you're much more datable. In one survey of 554 undergrads, researchers found that overweight women were less likely to date than their peers. What's more, you're marriage material if you're thin. Research shows that overweight women are significantly less likely to marry than are women of average weight, particularly if they were overweight as young adults.

Losing weight can do wonders for your sex life too. Duke University researchers did a study of 187 extremely obese adults, who were asked about their sex lives before and after they lost weight. It turned out the proportion of women who did not feel sexually attractive fell from 68 percent before they began a weight loss program to 26 percent a year later. There were similar decreases in the percentages of women who didn't want to be seen naked, had little sexual drive, avoided sexual encounters, had difficulty with sexual performance or didn't enjoy sex. Among men, sex improved in most of the categories, but the improvements were less dramatic, probably because there are a lot more appearance-related pressures on women.

The romantic world revolves around physical appearances. If you want a love life with great sex, lose the weight.

Get Richer

Get in shape and you can improve your financial shape too. It's considerably more expensive to be unfit than it is to be fit, mainly because you're sicker more often and you pay higher medical bills. People who are overweight, and particularly those who are obese, are significantly more likely to have expensive-to-treat diseases like diabetes, heart disease and cancer.

And while I'm at it, did you know your employment prospects will improve after you lose weight? It's true! People with weight problems sometimes don't get hired. In the job market, appearance counts for a lot. Employers think fat people are lazy, incompetent, slow-moving and might have poor attendance. Studies have shown that fat people are paid less than employees of average weight.

I hate fat discrimination. It's wrong. But this is the world we live in. It's not going to change anytime soon, so get over it. Lose weight and you won't have to deal with it.

Thin people look better and, like it or not, get paid more. If you're trim and healthy, you don't have an absentee problem. You might even be more productive on the job. All of this helps your earning potential. So if you want to live well and make your mortgage or rent payment, get those pounds off.

(continued on page 18)

LEAN 17:   Are You Ready to Be a Total Hottie?

Take this quiz to see if you are ready to go on the 17 Day Diet. A successful and healthy weight loss requires the right frame of mind. Circle the answer that best describes your level of commitment.

1. When I think about starting the 17 Day Diet, I feel excited.

    A. Yes   **B.** Somewhat   **C.** Unsure   **D.** Not at all

2. I feel that weight loss and fitness are very important.

    A. Yes   **B.** Somewhat   **C.** Unsure   **D.** Not at all

3. I am determined to eat more healthfully.

    A. Yes   **B.** Somewhat   **C.** Unsure   **D.** Not at all

4. I want to look better and feel sexier.

    A. Yes   **B.** Somewhat   **C.** Unsure   **D.** Not at all

5. I am willing to follow the food plans in this book.

    A. Yes   **B.** Somewhat   **C.** Unsure   **D.** Not at all

6. I will eat more fruits and vegetables.

    A. Yes   **B.** Somewhat   **C.** Unsure   **D.** Not at all

7. I will give up soft drinks, candy and other sweets while following this diet.

    A. Yes   **B.** Somewhat   **C.** Unsure   **D.** Not at all

8. I will scale back on my alcohol intake.

    A. Yes   **B.** Somewhat   **C.** Unsure   **D.** Not at all

9. I will prepare more meals at home and eat out less frequently.

    A. Yes   **B.** Somewhat   **C.** Unsure   **D.** Not at all

10. I will increase my water intake.

    A. Yes   **B.** Somewhat   **C.** Unsure   **D.** Not at all

11. I am willing to cut back on starchy foods like white bread, pasta and sugary breakfast cereals.

   A. Yes   **B.** Somewhat   **C.** Unsure   **D.** Not at all

12. I feel confident that I can stick to this plan for at least 17 days.

   A. Yes   **B.** Somewhat   **C.** Unsure   **D.** Not at all

13. I will eat at least 3 meals and 1 snack a day.

   A. Yes   **B.** Somewhat   **C.** Unsure   **D.** Not at all

14. I will not make excuses to sabotage myself.

   A. Yes   **B.** Somewhat   **C.** Unsure   **D.** Not at all

15. I can commit to exercising at least 17 minutes a day.

   A. Yes   **B.** Somewhat   **C.** Unsure   **D.** Not at all

16. I want to change my eating and health habits for life.

   A. Yes   **B.** Somewhat   **C.** Unsure   **D.** Not at all

17. I understand how diet, obesity and chronic illnesses are linked.

   A. Yes   **B.** Somewhat   **C.** Unsure   **D.** Not at all

Scoring: Give yourself a 3 for each A answer; a 2 for each B answer; a 1 for each C answer; and a 0 for each D answer. Add up your score.

0 to 17 points: Immediately re-evaluate your commitment to improving your health. If you don't act decisively now, serious health problems are on the horizon.

18 to 26 points: Go back over your answers and see what you need to shore up. You may be taking some unnecessary risks with your health and should make an extra effort to change.

27 to 42 points: Re-examine your desire to go on the 17 Day Diet. What improvements can you make to boost your score? You need just a little bit more determination and commitment to *be thinner and healthier.*

43 to 51 points: You're ready to start the 17 Day Diet and enjoy success—congratulations!

If my message seems too in-your-face, I apologize for the delivery—but not for the content. I'm speaking out because I care. I just want you to get healthy and enjoy your life to the fullest.

You must believe you can do this. It doesn't matter how often you have failed in the past; your past does not equal your future. What matters now is focusing on what you want, identifying what you need to get it and taking action. Your health and happiness are important, so stand strong.

7 REASONS Not to Freak Out about Being Fat

One of my patients joked recently about the pluses of her plus size: "I can shoplift in my cleavage. And I don't have to ask my boyfriend, 'Do I look fat in this?' I do." That conversation got me thinking about some of the health advantages to being overweight. Although I don't recommend staying fat, there are some pluses to being a plus size. Here are seven ways in which some padding can tip the scales in your favor.

Stronger Bones
A little meat on your frame can ward off osteoporosis, a condition of fragile bones that's less likely to occur in overweight women. Weight-bearing bones stay stronger.

Healthier Hearts and Lower Risk of Diabetes
Women with larger thighs have a lower risk of heart disease and early death, says a study in the *British Medical Journal.* Those with stick-thin legs face the greatest chance of developing heart disease. Why? Added lower-body muscle mass can promote a better metabolism. Also, a 2008 study published in *Cell Metabolism* found that the fat that accumulates around the thighs and hips, called subcutaneous fat, actually lowers risk of diabetes. Pear shapes, be proud.

Glowing Skin

Recent twin studies have found that the sister with more weight was judged to have a more youthful look. A gaunt face can definitely add some years, so carrying an extra few pounds can help create a more youthful appearance. It may also help to fill out a few of those more significant wrinkles that scream out "aging!"

Bigger Boobs

The more you weigh, the bigger they get. Breasts are made up of mostly fat, and any excess pounds practically go straight to your chest. Unfortunately, when you lose weight, boob flab is one of the first things to go.

Increased Fertility

Are you thinking of starting—or growing—your family? Underweight women were 72 percent more likely to miscarry, reports a London study. More specifically, leaner women when they conceived had a much higher percentage of miscarrying within three months of pregnancy. However, those few extra pounds on overweight women actually proved to have the opposite effect on their pregnancy.

Faster Metabolism

It's not the skinny folks who have a fast metabolism; it's the over-weight people! It takes more energy to operate anything bigger, so bigger people use more energy to do the same things that smaller people do. But metabolism isn't the only thing that determines weight; it's also how much you eat and exercise that matters.

Best Reason of All

People who are really out of shape, who start exercising, get fitter faster! The fact is your body wants to be in shape. It wants to be healthy. It wants to look good. It wants to be hot! So, the more out of shape you are, the faster your body will respond to your weight-loss efforts.

Review

- The 17 Day Diet is a rapid weight-loss plan designed to produce satisfying, lasting weight loss.

- Most people can expect to lose up to 10 to 15 pounds during the first 17 days.

- Rapid weight-loss plans have been shown in research to be effective in helping people keep their weight off.

- The 17 Day Diet works by improving digestive and metabolic health.

- The 17 Day Diet is organized into 4 Cycles, each working together to help your body reach its ideal weight and stabilize there.

- Stay upbeat and positive. No matter what you weigh right now, stop beating yourself up over it. So much in your life can change for the better: your figure, health, relationships, financial stability and more.

2

Burn, Baby, Burn

....

ere's the part of the book in which I talk about how the
17 Day Diet works. Don't worry. I won't lapse into any mind-
numbing "doctor speak." You know, medical terms that sound
scarier than the disease, like cephalalgia (headache) or pneumonitis
(lung inflammation). Most people have no idea what their doctors are
saying. They could be giving them the latest medical research or the
recipe for chocolate cheesecake in Latin. They couldn't tell.

I make a real effort to explain things in everyday terms. Sometimes, it's hard. I used to try to explain blood tests to patients in five
minutes. It finally dawned on me that it took me eight years to understand this stuff, so I can't expect anyone to comprehend it during one
office visit. You don't need to study medical books to understand what
doctors say anyway; just watch TV shows and movies.

Back to the topic of dieting: let me insert Rita's story here. If the
subject of weight loss came up in conversation, she'd walk away. About
25 pounds overweight, Rita was deep-down scared that she could get
heavier if she didn't do something. But she just wasn't ready to con-
front the issue head-on. The idea of dieting and taking weight off

21

slowly was frustrating, so she kept putting it off. But the 17 Day Diet appealed to her. It sounded doable and quick—it is. Rita decided to give it a try.

Here's what she said: "I can't believe how well the 17 Day Diet works. I lost 10 pounds the first 17 days, and I feel so energetic. What gives? How does it work?"

Basically, Rita was hooked (in a positive way) and has used the diet to get to her goal and stay there. She stayed motivated.

I explained to Rita that for a diet and exercise program to be successful, it must be safe, easy to follow and easy to stick to. It must have a certain balance of nutrients to activate fat-burning. It must generate results in a reasonable period of time. And it must help initiate a pattern of healthy habits that lead to lifelong weight control. The 17 Day Diet can help you accomplish all of this and more. What follows is a careful look at the elements that make this diet work.

What Do You Get to Eat on the 17 Day Diet?

First let me say, nutrition is too confusing, even for doctors. Everything is either good or bad for you. And that can change from moment to moment each time a new bit of research is unveiled. Broccoli may double your life span this week, but next week it might be the end of you.

Several years ago, blueberries became the fruit of choice, being touted as the answer for everything from rejuvenating your brain to inhibiting the growth of cancer cells. Now they're being added to cosmetics. If they can prevent your brain from aging, why not put them in a skin cream? Maybe blueberries can stop wrinkles too.

I think you have to be living under a rock not to know that lean proteins, fruits, vegetables and small amounts of grains are naturally good for you. The 17 Day Diet is based on those foods. That's one reason why the diet isn't a fad; it's based on really healthy foods, the stuff we should all be eating anyway, but aren't.

With these wonderful foods, we get the body to store the good (health-building nutrients) and expel the bad (fat and toxins) by retraining your digestive system and your metabolism.

Many long and informative books have been written about nutrition and how it works in the body. For the purpose of this book, I'll explain what you need to know about the nutrients your body needs to lose weight, and I'll do it in the clearest, most basic terms.

Enjoy Plenty of Protein

The 17 Day Diet is generous in protein. But I don't mean 27 eggs and 18 strips of bacon washed down with the drippings. I mean lean foods such as chicken, fish, lean meats and other protein-rich foods.

Protein is a powerful fat torcher—for six reasons:

1. Digesting protein takes more energy (calories) than digesting carbs or fat does; thus, your body burns a few extra calories after eating protein.

2. Including ample protein in your diet spurs one of your body's fat-burning mechanisms: the production of the hormone glucagon. Glucagon signals your body to move dietary fat into your bloodstream and use it for energy rather than just store it.

3. Consuming enough protein helps you preserve lean muscle mass that might otherwise be sacrificed on a rapid weight-loss diet. Of course, the more lean muscle you have, the more calories you burn, even at rest.

4. Eating protein helps keep your blood sugar on an even keel, so you don't get the shakes or drops in energy.

5. Having enough protein in your diet boosts your metabolism, and it does this by stepping up the action of your thyroid gland. (One of the main duties of the thyroid is to regulate metabolism.)

6. Including protein with meals helps tame your appetite so that you don't stuff yourself.

Venture into Vegetables

If you haven't eaten vegetables since you were 11, let's spend a second on this "I hate vegetables" thing.

You hate all vegetables? There isn't one you like, no matter how it's prepared? If you eliminate all vegetables from your diet, you're giving up some very important nutrients and really narrowing your food options. Vegetables are loaded with fiber, vitamins and minerals. Shunning them is a bad idea. Why not learn to prepare them WITH herbs and spices to satisfy your taste?

Pardon my assumption, but I think you, like thousands of other people I've talked to, believe that to lose weight, you have to subsist on carrot and celery sticks. But the old "carry around some celery sticks to munch on" mentality is gone forever. Aren't you relieved?

There are hundreds of different vegetables you can eat, even if you have to hide them in soups or spaghetti sauce. And you can pretty much eat your way through a couple of bushels without gaining any weight. If you want to change your body and get leaner, stronger and healthier, you have to eat vegetables. A March 1999 study conducted by the Energy Metabolism Laboratory at Tufts University found that the dieters who ate the widest variety of vegetables had the least amount of body fat. You need to eat vegetables if you want to get thin. Vegetables = thin. No vegetables = flabby.

Many of my patients have actually acquired a taste for fresh green leaves with cucumbers, tomatoes, red onions, carrots, mushrooms and all sorts of veggies. Some of them have even turned themselves into health nuts who only dip their forks into the salad dressing to really slash caloric intake.

There are more benefits. Eat more vegetables and you will:

- Bubble with energy all day.

- Improve your digestion and elimination, because veggies are high in fiber. High-fiber foods control appetite and help prevent excess calories from being stored as fat.

- Have glowing skin. Your skin loves vitamins and minerals, and you get most of those nutrients from veggies.

- Help prevent major killers like cancer and heart disease, because veggies are rich in disease-fighting antioxidants.

So yes, you heard me: eat your vegetables!

Forgo High-Sugar Fruits

Fruit may seem like a friendly diet food because it's low-fat, but here's an example of how having too much of a good thing can sabotage your diet. Certain fruits like pineapple, watermelon and bananas are high in sugar, and they don't promote fat loss. Too much sugar from any source can goad your body into converting more of what you eat into thigh-padding pounds.

I'm not going to ask you to shun all fruit. Just be moderate in how much you eat—two servings a day, only. On the first two Cycles of the 17 Day Diet, you'll stick to berries, apples, oranges and grapefruit, which are lower in sugar. When you eat like this, a fruit tooth will replace the sweet one that rules your mouth.

Curb the Carbs

Carbohydrates are energy foods. Without them, you'd get fuzzy headed, cranky and very tired, and no one would want to be around you. The low-carb diet craze deemed all carbs evil and fattening. People abandoned all forms of fruit, rice and pasta and ate mostly protein. The problem is, you can only eat so much protein and fat before you start to get nauseated by it.

Yet, not all carbs are the same. There are bad ones—stuff made mostly out of sugar or over-refined like white bread, white rice and white pasta. Sugar and sweets are the worst. Consider this: we are eating over twelve times the amount of sugar our great-grandparents consumed. That's roughly equivalent to 160 pounds of sugar per person per year. Now, imagine filling up your living room or garage with 160 of those one-pound packages you buy at the grocery store. Really get a mental picture of it. Let's say you don't eat as much as others, and cut it in half. It's still a hefty pile, isn't it? You see, most people have no idea that they're eating so much sugar. Much of it is hidden in processed, packaged foods we eat, as well as in beverages.

Depending on which Cycle you are in on the 17 Day Diet, you get to eat good carbs: fruit, vegetables, whole grains—anything that hasn't been stripped of its nutrition.

So the type of carbs you eat is important. But so is the amount. You can go overboard on carbs, even the good kind, and this can be devastating to your natural metabolic processes. Therefore, the 17 Day Diet is low-to-moderate in carbohydrates.

Many people are walking around completely unaware that they may be "carbohydrate sensitive." When you get carbohydrate sensitive, your body can no longer burn fat effectively, and a good deal of the carbohydrates you eat are packed away as fat. Carbohydrate sensitivity occurs when:

- You habitually eat too much sugar and refined carbohydrates (crackers, bagels, pasta, sugary cereals and desserts, white rice and white bread). Unfortunately, this sensitivity increases with age. It can also lead to insulin resistance, a condition just shy of type 2

CHECKUP: Are You Carbohydrate Sensitive?

Read through the statements below and circle "yes" or "no" depending on which response fits you best.

1. I crave carbohydrates and sugary foods much of the time. **Yes**   **No**

2. I have been overweight for much of my life and have struggled to lose weight   **Yes**   **No**

3. I am a woman and over forty.   **Yes**   **No**

4. I suffer from chronic or bouts of depression and compulsive overeating.   **Yes**   **No**

5. I sometimes suffer from nervousness or irritability.   **Yes**   **No**

6. When I eat sugar, I get tired and groggy, and I don't think as clearly.   **Yes**   **No**

7. I reach for carbohydrates rather than protein most or all of the time.   **Yes**   **No**

8. My diet consists of a lot of processed foods like white bread, pastas, sweets or sugary cereals.   **Yes**   **No**

9. I don't exercise very much or at all.   **Yes**   **No**

If you answered "yes" to three or more statements, you may be carbohydrate sensitive. Following the 17 Day Diet will help you by gradually reintroducing good carbs into your diet through each Cycle. Beans and lentils (legumes) do not raise blood sugar or insulin. Starchy vegetables, such as squash, corn, peas and yams, and fruits, such as oranges and apples, are also good and should be okay. So are brown rice, yams, oatmeal and other high-fiber cereals. Limit your servings to no more than two a day. More on this in Cycle 3.

diabetes. In insulin resistance, cells don't recognize glucose anymore, so glucose is barred from entering cells for energy. Your blood sugar tends to rise, you are more fatigued, and you gain more weight mostly around your waist and chest area.

- You suffer from chronic stress. Our bodies deal with stress by raising levels of cortisol, a hormone secreted from our adrenal glands. This, in turn, triggers the over-release of glucose and insulin into the bloodstream. The result is insulin resistance. To your physiology, being under chronic stress is the same as if you ate cake all day long.

- You're a woman. While men burn carbohydrates for energy, women tend to store them as fat. This is especially true as women age. Menopausal women are more prone. They don't have enough estrogen stores to deal with cortisol and its tendency to make the body store fat. Chalk it up to female biology.

Natural and unprocessed carbs are found in the 17 Day Diet in the vegetables and fruits allowed you. By Cycle 3, you'll get to introduce other carbs into the diet, including brown rice, oatmeal, whole grains, yams, potatoes, and other natural, high-fiber carbs.

Choose Fats That Burn Fat

Fat in the diet has been blamed for many modern lifestyle diseases: obesity, heart disease, cancer, diabetes and hypertension. Not all fats are created equal, however. Most people know by now they should limit intake of saturated fats, found in animal foods, and avoid trans fats entirely. Processed foods are loaded with trans fats.

Polyunsaturated fats, found mostly in fish and vegetable oils, are what I call "friendly fats." They are credited with keeping your skin supple and youthful, reducing harmful levels of cholesterol, lowering high blood pressure, contributing to brain and eye development and a host of other health benefits almost akin to a panacea. They also promote weight loss because they keep you feeling fuller for a longer period of time. This keeps you from eating too many calories.

Omega-3 fatty acids, found in fish, boost your metabolism. Adding some weekly servings of fish high in omega-3s (salmon, tuna, mackerel or sardines), while reducing calories, helped overweight people lose more weight than reducing calories alone, according to a study published in the *American Journal of Clinical Nutrition*. The researchers concluded that the omega-3s helped subjects burn more calories. If you don't like fish, take 3 grams of fish oil supplements daily.

Vitamins from Food

You're better off getting your vitamins from food. The body absorbs them more easily, and you'll just feel healthier. Required by your body in tiny amounts, vitamins play important roles in the metabolism of carbohydrates, proteins and fats. The vitamins you need daily are found in the 17 Day Diet as follows:

- *Vitamin A:* Green leafy vegetables, carrots, yams, fruits and eggs.
- *Vitamin B-complex:* Protein foods, whole grains, legumes, fruits and vegetables.
- *Vitamin C:* Fruits and vegetables.
- *Vitamin D:* Low-fat dairy foods, fish.
- *Vitamin E:* Whole grains, green leafy vegetables and eggs.

There's nothing wrong with taking a multivitamin-mineral pill daily. Like a lot of doctors, I recommend to adults that they take Flintstones vitamins—two a day. But no more than that, or you'll find yourself trying to stop your car with your bare feet.

Mighty Minerals

Minerals are among the heaviest substances ever, second only to Orson Welles. But of course, minerals don't make you heavy. They help you get thin, especially calcium, which may speed up the rate at which your body burns fat.

MISTER MD, CAN YOU PLEASE TELL ME ?

Are there natural supplements I can take instead of drugs to help lower my cholesterol?

Yes! A strict diet can probably reduce your cholesterol by 10 to 15 percent. Most docs agree that diet works best when combined with cholesterol-reducing drugs like statin drugs. Statins can drop LDL and total cholesterol by as much as a third by inhibiting the production of cholesterol by the liver. But these drugs come with a slew of potential side effects. The most common side effect is muscle aches. Other complaints include headaches, nausea, weakness, upset stomach and joint pain. I see these problems all the time.

Here's what I do for patients who can't tolerate statins but need to lower their cholesterol. I prescribe a combination of niacin (a B vitamin), fish oil and flaxseed oil in these amounts:

- **Niacin:** 250 milligrams a day for two or more weeks until they experience no flushing, which is a common side effect of niacin. After two weeks, I increase their dose to 500 milligrams a day. Once they tolerate that dose well, I increase the dose again to 750 milligrams daily.

- **Fish oil:** 3 grams a day.

- **Flaxseed oil:** 1 tablespoon a day (this can be part of a salad dressing).

All three substances are natural supplements you can purchase at a health food store or your pharmacy. The combination works powerfully to lower cholesterol, but always check with your own physician before self-medicating with supplements.

Like vitamins, minerals play a role in metabolism. But a major difference between the two nutrients is that minerals are constituents of bodily structures, such as bone, cartilage, and teeth, providing their hardness and strength. While vitamins help manufacture these structures, they do not become part of the structures themselves.

The minerals you need daily are found in the 17 Day Diet as follows:

Iron: Meats, poultry, eggs, green leafy vegetables and fruits.

Calcium: Yogurt, salmon, green leafy vegetables and broccoli.

Copper: Meats, shellfish.

Magnesium: Meats.

Phosphorus: Meats, poultry, fish.

Potassium: Fruits and vegetables.

Selenium: Whole grains, fish and eggs.

Zinc: Shellfish, meats, whole grains and vegetables.

The Benefits of Bugs

Not the kind you swat, spray or stomp, but the friendly bacteria called probiotics that live in your intestinal tract (hereafter referred to as your gut). You have a hundred trillion bacteria in your gut—ten times the number of cells—across three hundred to five hundred different species, and two hundred of these species can be lethal. This makes us more microbe than man. So you need to make sure you have enough of the good bacteria to ward off the bad.

There are actually two processes going on here. One is that the good bacteria help your intestinal wall construct a barrier against the bad bacteria. The second is that the good bacteria are like hostage negotiators you see on TV. They talk to the bad bacteria to keep them from starting a fight. The bad bacteria know the good guys mean business, so they drop their weapons and wave white flags.

The good guys do even more: probiotics may help people lose weight, according to lots of new research that adds to emerging evidence that part of the obesity problem might be an imbalance of bacteria in the gut.

Scientists are still exploring why, but many experts believe that people with certain communities of gut microbes may get more calories from their food and therefore pack on more fat than people with a different set of bugs. If you have a set of very, very efficient bacteria, they're going to extract every last bit of energy (calories) from what you eat. Manipulating these bacteria by diet or medications, you'd change how many calories you absorb. This may eventually become one approach to fighting obesity.

On the 17 Day Diet you'll enjoy foods that contain probiotics. These foods help your body digest foods and extract calories. Some types of probiotic foods include yogurt, kefir, miso and tempeh.

Fluid Assets

While following the 17 Day Diet, you should drink eight 8-ounce glasses of pure water daily. Drinking this amount of water is essential to weight loss.

First, it just takes up so much space in your tummy that you don't feel like eating much.

Second, water also helps your body metabolize stored fat. Your kidneys can't function properly without enough water. When kidneys don't work to capacity, some of their work is dumped onto the liver. One of the liver's primary functions is to metabolize stored fat into usable energy for the body, but if the liver has to do some of the kidneys' work, it can't operate at full capacity. As a result, it metabolizes less fat and more fat remains stored in the body, and weight loss stops.

> ### BEWARE: Negative Water
>
> The following fluids, which I call negative water, do not count toward your must-have daily allotment of water.
>
> Coffee*
>
> Tea*
>
> Diet sodas*
>
> Regular soda
>
> Energy drinks
>
> Juice
>
> Sports drinks (dilute with water—½ water and ½ sports drink
> if you are an athlete and use these products)
>
> Flavored waters
>
> *Coffee and tea are allowed on the 17 Day Diet, but do not count toward your 8 glasses of water.

Water also helps the body get rid of waste during weight loss. During weight loss, the body has a lot more waste to get rid of, and water helps flush it out.

Surprisingly, drinking an ample amount of water is the best treatment for fluid retention. When the body gets less water, it perceives this as a threat to survival and begins to hold on to every drop. Water is then stored outside the cells. This causes swollen feet, legs and hands. The best way to overcome the problem of water retention is to give your body what it needs: plenty of water. Only then will stored water be released.

So drink up. Before long, you'll be the skinniest person in the bathroom.

Special Mention Fluids: Green Tea and Coffee

For added fat-loss benefits, another beverage of choice is green tea, although it is technically a negative water. Certain natural chemicals

MISTER MD, CAN YOU PLEASE TELL ME ?

Am I allowed to drink alcohol on the 17 Day Diet?

I knew you'd ask that. Alcohol can actually be good for you. Major studies have concluded that moderate alcohol consumption cuts heart attack risk in half, largely because drinkers have about 15 percent higher levels of HDL cholesterol than nondrinkers, which prevents heart disease by cleansing the blood vessels of fatty buildups. Moderate alcohol means one drink a day: 5 ounces of wine, 12 ounces of beer or 1½ ounces of hard liquor.

Although a little alcohol is good for your heart, it's not that good for your waistline. Alcohol is dehydrating and interferes with fat-burning. The liver works overtime to metabolize the alcohol, so its job of burning fat gets less priority.

Once you get to Cycle 3, it's fine with me if you have one drink a day. Now, I don't recommend keeping it at your desk (at least for daytime use), but I do recommend it, especially red wine. One of my hobbies outside of work is enjoying fine red wine. To pursue my passion for drinking and collecting fine red wine, I enjoy attending wine tastings with my friends.

Red wine contains resveratrol (a powerful antioxidant found in grape skin). It turns off a gene for certain inflammatory proteins. These proteins ride around in your bloodstream. When there's a foreign body, like a toxic molecule from an infection or a toxin, the proteins attach it to your arterial wall. This attachment stimulates inflammation. Inflammation can lead to clogged arteries, blood clots, impotence and even a heart attack or stroke. One glass of red wine a day may help prevent these things. So, cheers.

called catechins in green tea increase fat-burning and stimulate thermogenesis, the calorie-burning process that occurs as a result of digesting and metabolizing food.

Green tea is also one of the foods that may block angiogenesis (sorry, I have to slip one technical term in here). Angiogenesis refers to a process of blood vessel growth. For example, angiogenesis that builds up a blood supply to tumors can unfortunately make the tumors grow. Scientists have discovered that angiogenesis does the same thing with fat tissue: It creates a blood supply to fat tissue too, so it can grow. Fat tissue and cancer feed on oxygen delivered by these new blood vessels.

There's excellent science published in the best journals that something in green tea inhibits angiogenesis. The jury is still out on all this, but until we know more, I suggest drinking three cups of green tea a day.

Although doctors should set an example, I confess I'm not much of a green tea drinker. If I'm having a cup, I'm probably in an Asian restaurant. I promise to do better, though, and drink more green tea.

Coffee is also permitted on the 17 Day Diet. The caffeine kicks your metabolism into high gear. Caffeine also jump-starts the breakdown of fat in the body. One to two cups a day is ideal.

How Much Should You Weigh?

As you begin the 17 Day Diet, have a specific weight goal in mind. In other words, shoot for a weight at which you feel you will look your best. Keep in mind that there's really no such thing as the "perfect" weight because we all come in a variety of body shapes, heights and bone structures. There are, however, "ideal weight ranges," so there is a simple equation I tend to follow:

If you're a woman: Take 100 pounds for the first five feet of your height, and add five pounds for each extra inch to get the midpoint of what should be your ideal body weight range. Then you need to factor in your body structure. Some people are smaller boned; others are big boned. If you're small boned, I subtract 15 percent from the normal-frame weights; if you're large boned, I add 15 percent to the normal-frame weights. For a lot of people, that's too much math. So I did the math for you:

WOMEN		
Small-Boned Frame	**Midpoint**	**Large-Boned Frame**
5' = 85	5' = 100	5' = 115
5' 1" = 90	5' 1" = 105	5' 1" = 121
5' 2" = 94	5' 2" = 110	5' 2" = 127
5' 3" = 98	5' 3" = 115	5' 3" = 132
5' 4" = 102	5' 4" = 120	5' 4" = 137
5' 5" = 106	5' 5" = 125	5' 5" = 144
5' 6" = 110	5' 6" = 130	5' 6" = 150
5' 7" = 115	5' 7" = 135	5' 7" = 155
5' 8" = 119	5' 8" = 140	5' 8" = 161
5' 9" = 123	5' 9" = 145	5' 9" = 167
5' 10" = 128	5' 10" = 150	5' 10" = 173
5' 11" = 132	5' 11" = 155	5' 11" = 178
6' = 136	6' = 160	6' = 184

If you're a man: Take 110 pounds for the first five feet of your height, and add six pounds for each extra inch to get the midpoint of what should be your ideal body weight range. Allow for being small or large boned, as explained above.

How Often Should You Weigh Yourself?

Not too many people like to weigh themselves. Doctors know this. After patients step on the scale, they think it is giving them the weight of a completely different person, like Hulk Hogan. Since we won't let them weigh naked, they tell us to subtract two pounds for their shoes, one pound for jewelry and three pounds if it is after the Big Mac and fries they had for lunch. Some people strip off this stuff faster than a Lexus left on a city side street at midnight and step on the scale again. But doctors' scales do not lie. Patients have to accept the truth. Their bodies, without consulting them, have been converting doughnuts, pizza and ice cream into fat.

Let's talk about scales for a moment. Your bathroom scale can be

SCIENCE SAYS: Use Your Brain to Get Buff

Medical studies have shown that visualizing yourself in the shape you want to be in can help you attain a trim, toned physique. The brain thinks very much in pictures. If you can call up a picture in your mind, you have a powerful way of making it happen. So it's important to get the image of your perfect body in your mind so you can create it.

Start imagining what your life will be like as a thin, healthy person. You'll be able to play, be active, really live, and enjoy living for your family. You'll be able to shop at normal stores, not own plus-sized clothes, and forget worrying about fitting into airplane seats. You'll no longer be a target of jokes or have people judge you. And you won't have to fear a future of diabetes, heart attack, stroke or other weight-related health issues. All of these images give your mind realistic goals to work toward.

a top tool for losing weight. I know, some people say throw it out. But those people are naturally thin or possibly teach aerobics classes. They don't need a scale.

If you skirt the scale, your weight might start going up, and you won't know it. Then, when the nurse forces you at pen point to ascend the scale at your next doctor's appointment and 302 pops up, you might go into shock.

Tracking your weight is one of the most important things you can do to prevent that from happening. It's also a habit that has helped people in the National Weight Control Registry—a group of several thousand "successful losers"—hold their weight steady. Registry participants have lost at least 30 pounds and kept it off for at least a year.

Yes, other things can tell you a lot about your weight: the way your clothes fit, how winded you feel going up a flight of stairs or how you look in the mirror. But weigh yourself too, every several days, or at least once a week, and definitely after each 17 Day Cycle.

Just resist weighing yourself dozens of times a day in hopes of a better outcome.

So take that candy jar off your desk. It may make you less popular with your co-workers, but you're on your way to a lighter life. And that's exciting.

LEAN 17: Facts about Fat

1. The average adult has 40 billion fat cells.

2. Fat is also one of the most abundant types of tissue in the body.

3. Fat tissue is a dynamic, complex and necessary component of life.

4. Girls are born with more fat cells than boys.

5. By the time you're a teenager, you will likely have all the fat cells you are ever going to have.

6. Fat grows when existing cells enlarge and when new cells get created.

7. The number of fat cells can go up, but not down.

8. When you lose weight, existing fat cells shrink.

9. Fat cells die, but your body quickly replenishes them with the same number.

10. Fat cells are bigger in obese people.

11. Fat cells come in two types: white and brown. White is the kind that makes your jeans too tight. Brown fat is found in babies and has the ability to burn energy.

12. Fat cells, like cancer cells and other cells in the body, feed themselves oxygen with new blood vessels in a process known as angiogenesis. Fat can't expand without expanding its blood vessels, just like a city can't expand without expanding its roads. Researchers are studying whether certain cancer drugs can starve fat cells to stop fat expansion the same way they starve tumors.

13. When you exercise, cells produce an enzyme that tells fatty tissue to release its stores for muscles to burn.

14. The liver stores glucose from food as glycogen and releases it into the bloodstream when energy is needed. Once glucose runs out, the body starts to burn fat.

15. Fat cells secrete estrogen, which is linked to certain types of cancer, chiefly breast cancer in postmenopausal women.

16. Body fat accumulates from head to toe and comes off the same way.

17. Body fat is like a ski suit: it provides insulation against the cold. A downside of getting thin is that you might shiver more often.

Review

- On the 17 Day Diet, you eat healthy foods: lean proteins, vegetables, low-sugar fruits, natural carbs, probiotics and friendly fats. These foods work together to improve your digestion and metabolism.

- The 17 Day Diet supplies the nutrients you need for good health.

- The 17 Day Diet limits carbs somewhat, because many people are carbohydrate sensitive, a condition that interferes with weight loss.

- Drinking water is vital for weight loss; so is drinking green tea.

3

Cycle 1:
Accelerate

· ·

Dropping up to 10 or 12 pounds over the next 17 days is possible, and you can see impressive results quickly if you follow to the letter Cycle 1: Accelerate.

The trouble with most diets (besides the boring food lists and the inevitable hunger pangs) is that it's tricky to find one that helps you shed pounds quickly without compromising the nutritional quality of your meals—and ultimately your health and vitality. This Cycle gets you on the road to lean quickly, plus keeps you full, energetic and motivated.

On this Cycle you can eat unlimited protein—including meat, poultry, eggs and fish, as well as many vegetables. But you limit your carbohydrate intake by initially cutting out white bread, potatoes, pasta, rice, chocolate, biscuits and sugary desserts and sweets. Fruit and fats are not banned, and that's good because both will add sweetness and flavor to your diet.

Cycle 1 is called Accelerate because its purpose is to trigger rapid weight loss in a healthy manner by mobilizing fat stores and flushing water and toxins from your system. The following are the things the Accelerate Cycle will be doing for you:

- Reducing carbohydrate intake slightly so that your body taps into its storage fat.

- Increasing protein intake so that your body goes into a fat-burning mode.

- Correcting improper digestion—a situation that can hold you back from fat-burning.

- Providing rapid weight loss at the start, so that you have the incentive to keep going.

- Getting out sugar, sweets, refined carbohydrates and other substances that cause those dreaded spikes and dips in blood sugar. Once you've broken that cycle, your body will simply not crave them anymore. In this Cycle, you're removing foods that don't work well for your body.

SCIENCE SAYS: Toxins and Metabolic Rate

I wouldn't be surprised if our livers went around saying: "I don't get no respect!" Day in and day out, we're exposed to toxins through drinking water, some foods and other sources. The liver, the primary organ of metabolism, has to work overtime to detoxify these things out of the body. Also, these particular toxins are stored in your fat cells—so as you start to shed pounds, they're released into your bloodstream.

A team of Quebec researchers found that when toxins are released while overweight people are dieting, their metabolic rate—the speed at which calories are burned—slows down considerably, even more than the slowdown often caused by dieting. Fortunately, many of the foods, particularly fruits and vegetables, on the 17 Day Diet are heroes at cleansing the body of toxins.

Source: *American Journal of Physiology—Regulatory, Integrative and Comparative Physiology,* 2001.

- Clearing your body of possible toxins. Pollutants in the body interfere with both the thyroid gland, which helps regulate the body's metabolism, and individual cells' energy factories (mitochondria), which convert fuel into energy.

If you reach your goal in the first 17 days, you can go right on to Cycle 4, maintenance. If you still have more weight to lose, move on to Cycle 2: Activate—and enjoy even more foods for another 17 days. And then it's on to Cycle 3 for the next 17 days, a more liberal version of the first two Cycles. And if you're waiting for the day when I declare that cupcakes are part of your diet, that day arrives with Cycle 4, designed to keep your weight off with the reintroduction of your favorite foods back into your life.

The Accelerate Cycle is the handiest diet tool you've got for getting—and keeping—your weight down. Look, if your diet goes AWOL for whatever reason—and you gain some weight back, you can always return to the Accelerate Cycle to get back on track. Do this and you'll keep getting closer to your ideal weight. It's a short-term strategy that will guarantee long-term results.

My Hunger/Fullness Meter

Your parents probably drilled into you that you were not allowed to leave the table unless you finished everything on your plate. That was good advice when portions were smaller, and everyone hated to waste food.

These days, most of us don't know when we're hungry and when we're full. We lose this ability by the time we reach kindergarten. And it's making us fat.

I have a solution: Dr. Mike's Hunger/Fullness Meter. The Fullness Meter is kind of like the "pain scale" doctors ask you about when you are in the hospital. Basically, you rate your hunger and fullness on a scale. This is not a new idea; there are lots of hunger scales out there. But the problem with most is that they want you to rate your hunger on a scale of 0 to 10. That's too complicated. What is the difference between a 0 or a 1, or a 9 or a 10, anyway? You'd spend so much time trying to figure out your rating that you won't have time to eat.

I say it's simpler to use a hunger rating from 1 to 2, and a fullness rating from 3 to 4. Here's how mine works.

Hunger Meter

1. **I'm a little hungry; my stomach feels as hollow as the promises of a politician.**
   Eat now to prevent yourself from progressing to 2. Other leading indicators of mild hunger are slight stomach growling, mild headache, shakiness and loss of concentration. If you aren't sure whether you're actually hungry, you're probably not. You may be confusing true hunger with boredom, fatigue or thirst.

2. **I'm so hungry I could eat the lining of an empty Spam can. My stomach is growling so loud it scared off a junkyard dog. I've got to get something to eat, and fast.**
   Don't let yourself get here. You'll be eating a package of Twinkies and guzzling Coke like crazy.

Fullness Meter

3. **I'm starting to feel full. I will stop now so that I can save on my grocery bill.**
   You have entered that pleasant zone where you are no longer hungry but not quite full, either. Feel honorable about leaving a little room in your stomach. Try to keep yourself here at meals, never starving, never stuffed.

4. **I'm so stuffed I'll have to waddle over to the couch to collapse.**
   You have eaten too much, even if it's all on your diet. Avoid this

extreme; practice more restraint. Don't feel obligated to clean your plate, either. Stop eating as soon as your stomach feels full. Those extra bites of food that you're trying not to waste add unneeded calories.

As you go through your day and manage your mealtimes, ask yourself how hungry or full you are, based on my Hunger/Fullness Meter. Your goal is to listen to your body and let go of external cues, such as the clock, to tell you when, and how much, to eat.

General Guidelines for the Accelerate Cycle

1. Follow the Accelerate Cycle for 17 days. If you reach your weight-loss goal, move on to Cycle 4: Arrive. If you have more weight to lose, go on to the next Cycle: Activate.

2. Your diet will consist of lean proteins, vegetables, low-sugar fruits, probiotic foods like yogurt, and good fats. Starchy foods such as potatoes, legumes, brown rice, corn and oatmeal are not permitted on this Cycle.

3. Remove skin from chicken or turkey prior to cooking or purchase skinless poultry.

4. About eggs: You may eat up to two eggs a day. But stick to no more than four yolks per week if your physician has diagnosed you with high cholesterol. Egg whites can be eaten without restriction.

5. Enjoy fresh vegetables and fruits as much as possible. For convenience, frozen and canned items are fine, if chosen in moderation. They must be unsweetened, however.

6. Do not eat any fruit after 2:00 p.m. Fruit is a carb. The timing of carbohydrate intake is very important. I've found that carbs eaten early in the day supply the body with only enough

fuel (in the form of glycogen stored in muscles) to energize the body the rest of the day. You'll find that this approach also improves your waistline. If you eat carbs in the evening, it's harder for the body to burn them off because you expend less energy in the evening. Those carbs might be stored as fat.

7. Avoid alcohol and sugar in order to help your body eliminate toxins, improve digestion and burn fat.

8. Adopt the habit of drinking green tea. It contains some caffeine but offers compounds that help burn fat.

9. About probiotic foods: Research indicates that they boost the immune system and promote gut-cleansing bacteria. Probiotic foods are also thought to help the body burn fat. If you don't like yogurt, try the sugar-free fruit-flavored yogurt or cultured milk, such as low-fat acidophilus milk (it tastes just like regular low-fat milk). Also, you can still get the friendly bacteria you need. Most health food stores sell capsules containing probiotics; follow the manufacturer's instructions for dosage.

10. Eat slowly and only until full; do not overload your stomach.

11. Drink eight 8-ounce glasses of pure water a day.

12. Exercise at least 17 minutes a day.

Take It Off: The Accelerate Cycle Food List

Lean Proteins

Here's where you'll be getting a lot of your fat-burning power. Eat all you want of the following proteins. They're freebies. The 17 Day Diet is purposely high in protein because it stimulates the reduction of body fat.

Fish*

Salmon, canned or fresh

Sole

Flounder

Catfish

Tilapia

Canned light tuna (in water)

*Opt for wild-caught rather than farm-raised fish, which may have received
doses of antibiotics. Avoid the bigger fish such as swordfish, shark, king
mackerel and albacore tuna. They are the most likely to carry metals like
methyl-mercury, which is considered a toxin.

Poultry

Chicken breasts

Turkey breasts

Ground turkey, lean

Eggs (2 eggs = 1 serving)

Egg whites (4 egg whites = 1 serving)

Cleansing Vegetables

Eat all you want from the following list. They're freebies too. I call
these cleansing vegetables because they support detoxification in the
intestines, blood and liver, and offer protective antioxidants. A few
honorable mentions:

Cauliflower, cabbage, broccoli, and Brussels sprouts supply
important phytochemicals (disease-fighting substances in
plants), which help the liver detoxify chemicals, drugs and
pollutants.

Asparagus, spinach and okra are all notable sources of glutathi-
one, a vital compound that aids in the removal of fat-soluble
toxins. (So is cooked chicken.)

LEAN 17: Maximize the Health Power of Fruits and Veggies

1. Look for fresh produce that is crisp and not wilted. Fresh = nutritious.

2. When buying fresh fruits, look for bruises on the fruit. Bruising initiates a chemical reaction that saps the nutrient content.

3. When purchasing salad-in-a-bag, look for a colorful medley of greens in the package. The more color, the more antioxidants and phytochemicals in the vegetables.

4. Always select the brightest, most colorful fruits and vegetables on the shelves. The brighter the color, the more vitamins and nutrients in the produce.

5. Go for darker shades of green when buying lettuce. Dark-leafed lettuce, like Romaine, is richer in certain B vitamins than are lighter varieties of lettuce such as iceberg.

6. Buy certain vegetables such as onions and sweet peppers in all their various colors for a greater array of nutrients.

7. Purchase fresh fruits and vegetables in season when their flavor and nutrition are at peak levels.

8. Buy locally grown fruit and vegetables when you can. They tend to be more nutrient-rich because they come picked right from the field. (A lot of nutrient loss occurs when produce is in transit for delivery to supermarkets.)

9. Berries are highly perishable. At the grocery store, look at the bottom of the container. Staining is a sign that the fruit has been bruised or is overripe. Nutrient loss has already set in, and the fruit will spoil rapidly.

10. Look for the brightest strawberries possible. A bright color signals exceptional nutrient quality. If berries show too much whiteness at their base, they're less nutritious.

11. Sniff berries to test for freshness. A pleasant aroma indicates good flavor, ripeness and nutritional goodness.

12. Buy a variety of fruits and vegetables on the food lists. The greater the variety of foods you eat, the healthier your nutrition.

13. Eat fruits and vegetables raw whenever possible. Generally, raw produce is healthier. Exception to the raw rule: Cooked carrots and tomatoes yield more antioxidants.

14. Cook vegetables the shortest time possible to preserve nutrients.

15. Steaming vegetables is a great way to keep nutrients from escaping.

16. Avoid thawing frozen fruits and vegetables prior to cooking. As foods thaw, microorganisms possibly present in food may begin to multiply, spoiling the food.

17. In most cases, avoid peeling. Nutrients and fiber are lost when produce is peeled.

Spinach, broccoli, tomatoes, and Brussels sprouts contribute alpha-lipoic acid, a powerful antioxidant that destroys harmful free radicals, which are byproducts of detoxification.

Onions accelerate the breakdown of fats in your food. As a result, your body is more apt to excrete them than to store them in fat cells.

Greens have diuretic properties (which help you lose water weight), and their ability to stabilize blood sugar prevents binge eating.

Artichokes have a range of health-promoting benefits. This veggie scores high on the antioxidant scale, thanks to the presence of cynarin and silymarin. These two phytochemicals are thought to lower cholesterol, protect liver cells from toxins, enhance circulation, and aid digestion. Both antioxidants are found in the leaves and the heart of the vegetable.

Artichoke

Artichoke hearts

Asparagus

Bell peppers, green, orange, red, yellow

Broccoli

Brussels sprouts

Cabbage

Carrots

Cauliflower

Celery

Cucumbers

Eggplant

Garlic

Green beans

Green, leafy vegetables (including beet greens, turnip greens, collard greens)

Kale

Leeks

Lettuce, all varieties

Mushrooms

Okra

Onions

Parsley

Scallions

Spinach

Tomatoes

Watercress

Low-Sugar Fruit—2 servings daily

Low-sugar fruits are good sources of fiber that provide bulk and digest slowly, helping you feel full. They're also full of water, high in fiber and super low in calories, which makes them ideal for weight loss.

Apples

Berries, all types

Grapefruit

Oranges

Peaches

Pears

Plums

Prickly pear cactus

Prunes

Red grapes

Probiotic Foods—2 servings daily

Probiotics help balance your digestive system, resulting in an overall increase in the efficiency of digestion. Research shows that probiotics may also help fight obesity. If you've been under stress, taken antibiotics or eaten a lot of foods packaged with preservatives, these things

MISTER MD, CAN YOU PLEASE TELL ME ?

What if I take a medicine that interacts with grapefruit?

Grapefruit and grapefruit juice (which you do not drink on the 17 Day Diet) interact with a few specific prescription drugs, and one is statins, taken to lower cholesterol. Grapefruit and grapefruit juice may prevent the liver from sufficiently breaking down the drug, resulting in a higher dose entering the bloodstream. Most doctors know this.

This interaction was discovered back in the 1990s with research studies. A handful of these studies talked about the "usual dose" of grapefruit juice. But the usual dose was sometimes a whole quart a day! No one drinks that much grapefruit juice, even if grapefruit juice is your favorite food.

Personally, I like grapefruit. I eat it for its taste, vitamin C and fiber. Plus, I like folding the grapefruit in half and squeezing the juice into a spoon.

What I tell my patients who take statins is that they may enjoy ½ grapefruit or 1 cup of grapefruit juice (no juice on the Accelerate Cycle of the 17 Day Diet, though) in the morning.

Secondly, I instruct them to always take their statins in the evening. These measures help minimize any grapefruit-drug interaction. And they still get to squeeze their grapefruit.

Before doing these things, you should make sure to consult with your own physician.

can kill off the beneficial bugs in your system—so eating more probiotic foods is a good idea.

There's no RDA for probiotics. To maintain health, a probiotic count of 5 to 10 billion is adequate. That may sound like a lot, but consider this: a 6 oz. serving of yogurt contains around 17 billion probiotics.

Yogurt, any type, including Greek-style, sugar-free fruit flavored; plain; and low-fat (6 oz. container = 1 serving)

Kefir: similar to a drinking-style yogurt; great for making smoothies (1 cup = 1 serving)

Low-fat acidophilus milk (1 cup = 1 serving)

Yakult (small 50-calorie bottle)

Breakstone LiveActive cottage cheese (½ cup = 1 serving)

Reduced salt miso dissolved in low-fat, low-sodium broth (1 tablespoon = 1 serving)

Tempeh (a fermented cake of pressed soybeans) (4 oz. = 1 serving)

Sauerkraut (½ cup = 1 serving)

Kimchi (Korean cabbage) (½ cup = 1 serving) Find it in Asian supermarkets or natural food stores, and enjoy a small amount as a side dish with meals.

Friendly Fats: 1 to 2 tablespoons daily

I don't purposely tell my patients to eat fats, unless it's the healthy kind such as fish oil, olive oil or flaxseed oil. These healthful fats can help reduce the risk of heart disease, stroke, certain cancers and diabetes, as well as promote joint health, prevent muscle loss and encourage fat loss and muscle toning.

Olive oil

Flaxseed oil

Condiments

Condiments and seasonings are allowed in moderation: salsa, low-carb marinara sauce, lite soy sauce, low-carb ketchup, fat-free sour cream, low-fat, low-sodium broth, Truvia (a non-caloric sweetener made from natural ingredients), sugar-free jams and jellies, vegetable cooking spray, fat-free cheeses (e.g. Parmesan), fat-free salad dressing, salt, pepper, vinegar, mustard, herbs and spices.

Meal Planning Made Easy

It's easy to remember what to eat during this Cycle:

- As much as you want of specific proteins and cleansing vegetables.

- Supplement these foods with 2 low-sugar fruits daily; 2 servings of probiotic foods such as yogurt, kefir, Yakult (small 50-calorie bottle), acidophilus milk, reduced salt miso dissolved in low-fat, low-sodium broth, sauerkraut (½-cup serving) and 1 to 2 table-spoons of friendly fat. It's that easy.

You do not have to count anything, except your 2 daily fruit servings, your 2 daily probiotic servings and your fat serving.

Here is a typical day on the Accelerate Cycle:

Breakfast

- 2 eggs or 4 egg whites, prepared without oil; or 1 serving probiotic food such as yogurt

- 1 fruit serving

- 1 cup green tea

MISTER MD, CAN YOU PLEASE TELL ME ?

Can I take a probiotic supplement instead of eating probiotic foods?

Yes. Probiotics come in supplement form that you can buy at your pharmacy or health food store. Look for a probiotic supplement that contains 10 to 20 billion colony-forming units (CFUs), and read the label to learn how it should be stored.

Lunch
- Liberal amounts of protein in the form of fish, poultry or eggs plus unlimited amounts of cleansing vegetables; or 1 probiotic serving plus unlimited amounts of cleansing vegetables
- 1 cup green tea

Dinner
- Liberal amounts of protein in the form of fish or chicken
- Unlimited amounts of cleansing vegetables
- 1 cup green tea

Snacks
- 2nd fruit serving
- 2nd probiotic serving

Additional
- 1 serving friendly fat (1 to 2 tablespoons to use on salads or vegetables or for cooking)

17 Sample Menus

Here are examples of how you can create your daily menu during the Accelerate Cycle. You may follow these exactly or create your own menus based on the above guidelines. Some days include easy-to-make recipes. You'll find these in Chapter 14.

Wake-up drink

Every morning, as soon as you rise, drink one 8-ounce cup of hot water. Squeeze half a lemon into the cup; the lemon stimulates your digestive juices. Your goal is to drink at least seven more glasses of water by the end of the day.

The rate at which you burn calories drops if you're dehydrated. And if you're dehydrated, your body doesn't absorb nutrients properly. "Negative waters" such as coffee or tea do not count toward your total daily fluid intake.

Consult your physician regarding the amount of your daily water intake if you have been diagnosed with congestive heart failure. Water requirements vary.

Day 1

Breakfast
- 2 scrambled egg whites
- ½ grapefruit, or other fresh fruit
- 1 cup green tea

Lunch
- Large green salad topped with tuna; drizzle with 1 tablespoon olive or flaxseed oil and 2 tablespoons balsamic vinegar
- 1 cup green tea

Dinner
- Plenty of grilled chicken with liberal amounts of any vegetables from the list, steamed or raw
- 1 cup green tea

Snacks
- 6 oz. sugar-free plain yogurt mixed with 1 to 2 tablespoons sugar-free jam or other probiotic serving
- 1 serving of fruit from the list

Day 2

Breakfast

- 6 oz. plain low-fat yogurt, mixed with 1 cup berries or other fruit (chopped) on the list. You may sweeten the mixture with 1 packet of Truvia or sugar-free fruit jam.
- 1 cup green tea

Lunch

- *Super Salad* (page 269)
- 1 cup green tea

Dinner

- Plenty of grilled or baked salmon with liberal amounts of any vegetables from the list, steamed or raw
- 1 cup green tea

Snacks

- 6 oz. sugar-free fruit-flavored yogurt or 1 cup plain low-fat yogurt, sweetened with Truvia or a tablespoon of sugar-free fruit jam
- 1 serving of fruit

Day 3

Breakfast

- 2 hard-boiled or poached eggs
- ½ grapefruit or other fresh fruit in season
- 1 cup green tea

Lunch

- 1 large bowl of *Chicken-Vegetable Soup* (page 273)
- 1 cup green tea

Dinner

- Plenty of roasted turkey breast or turkey tenderloin, steamed carrots and steamed asparagus
- 1 cup green tea

Snacks

- 6 oz. plain low-fat yogurt, sweetened with Truvia or a tablespoon of sugar-free fruit jam
- *Kefir Smoothie* (page 267)

Day 4

Breakfast

- *Kefir Smoothie* (page 267)
- 1 cup green tea

Lunch

- *Marinated Vegetable Salad* (page 273) or *Super Salad* (page 269)
- 6 oz. plain low-fat yogurt with a sliced fresh peach, or other fruit in season, for dessert
- 1 cup green tea

Dinner

- *Eggplant Parmesan* (page 274)
- Alternative dinner: Any of the lean proteins with plenty of cooked cleansing vegetables from the list
- 1 cup green tea

Day 5

Breakfast
- 2 scrambled egg whites
- ½ grapefruit or other fresh fruit in season
- 1 cup green tea

Lunch
- *Spinach Salad* (page 270)
- 1 cup green tea

Dinner
- Ground turkey patties, with side salad drizzled with 1 table-spoon olive or flaxseed oil and 2 tablespoons balsamic vinegar
- 1 cup green tea

Snacks
- 1 cup fresh berries
- 6 oz. plain low-fat yogurt, sweetened with Truvia or a tablespoon of sugar-free fruit jam

Day 6

Breakfast
- 6 oz. plain low-fat yogurt, mixed with 1 cup berries or other fruit (chopped) on the list. You may sweeten the mixture with 1 packet of Truvia or a tablespoon of sugar-free fruit jam.
- 1 cup green tea

Lunch

- *Lettuce Wraps* (page 272) or grilled chicken breast with tossed salad drizzled with 1 tablespoon olive or flaxseed oil and 2 tablespoons balsamic vinegar
- 1 cup green tea

Dinner

- *Sesame Fish*, or any grilled or baked fish
- Steamed cleansing vegetables
- 1 cup green tea

Snacks

- 2nd fruit serving of your choice
- 2nd probiotic serving of your choice

Day 7

Breakfast

- 2 scrambled eggs, 4 scrambled egg whites or 1 scrambled egg plus 2 scrambled egg whites. Top with salsa (optional).
- 1 apple or 1 cup fresh berries
- 1 cup green tea

Lunch

- *Taco Salad*
- 1 cup green tea

Dinner

- A stir-fry of vegetables (broccoli, onions, julienne carrots, red pepper, etc.) and chicken strips with 1 tablespoon olive oil. Season with a little garlic, ginger, and lite soy sauce.
- 1 cup green tea

Snacks

- 2nd fruit serving plus 1 probiotic serving of your choice
- 2nd probiotic serving of your choice

Day 8

Breakfast

- 6 oz. plain low-fat yogurt, mixed with 1 cup berries or other fruit (chopped) on the list. You may sweeten the mixture with 1 packet of Truvia or a tablespoon of sugar-free fruit jam.
- 1 cup green tea

Lunch

- Salmon salad: 2 cups salad vegetables (lettuce, tomatoes, onions, cucumbers, etc.), baked or canned salmon, drizzled with 1 table-spoon olive or flaxseed oil, mixed with 2 tablespoons balsamic vinegar and seasonings.
- 1 cup green tea

Dinner

- Turkey burger (made with lean ground turkey)
- Steamed vegetables (choose from list of cleansing vegetables)
- Side salad drizzled with 1 tablespoon olive or flaxseed oil, mixed with 2 tablespoons balsamic vinegar and seasonings
- 1 cup green tea

Snacks

- 2nd fruit serving
- 2nd probiotic serving

Day 9

Breakfast

- *Greek Egg Scramble* (page 268)
- 1 fresh orange
- 1 cup green tea

Lunch

- *Nicoise Salad* (page 269)
- 1 cup green tea

Dinner

- Grilled chicken breast (marinate in fat-free Italian dressing, then broil or grill)
- Steamed vegetables (choose from list of cleansing vegetables)
- 1 cup green tea

Snacks

- *Kefir Smoothie* (page 267)
- 2nd probiotic serving

Day 10

Breakfast

½ cup Breakstone LiveActive cottage cheese
1 medium pear, sliced
1 cup green tea

Lunch

Balsamic Artichoke (page 270; use non-fat salad dressing as a dipping sauce)
1 medium apple
1 cup green tea

Dinner

- *Oven Barbecued Chicken* (page 275)
- Side salad drizzled with 1 tablespoon olive or flaxseed oil, mixed with 2 tablespoons balsamic vinegar and seasonings
- 1 cup green tea

Snacks

- 2nd probiotic serving
- Raw, cut-up veggies

Day 11

Breakfast

- *Yogurt Fruitshake* (page 267)
- 1 cup green tea

Lunch

- *Super Salad* (page 269)
- 1 cup green tea

Dinner

- *Turkey Black Bean Chili* (page 276)
- Side salad drizzled with 1 tablespoon olive or flaxseed oil, mixed with 2 tablespoons balsamic vinegar and seasonings
- 1 cup green tea

Snacks

- 2 probiotic servings

Day 12

Breakfast

- 2 hard-boiled or poached eggs
- ½ grapefruit or other fresh fruit in season
- 1 cup green tea

Lunch

- Baked or grilled chicken breast
- Tomatoes—sliced or stewed
- 1 medium orange
- 1 cup green tea

Dinner

- Baked or grilled fish, any kind from the list
- Cleansing vegetables, as many from the list as you wish
- 1 cup green tea

Snacks

- *Kefir Smoothie* (page 267)
- 2nd probiotic food

Day 13

Breakfast

- *Kefir Smoothie* (page 267)
- 1 cup green tea

Lunch

- Tuna tossed with 1 tablespoon olive oil and a tablespoon of vinegar, served over a generous bed of lettuce
- 1 cup green tea

Dinner

- Plenty of roast turkey or chicken
- Tomato and onion salad, tossed with fat-free salad dressing
- 1 cup green tea

Snacks

- 2nd fruit serving
- 2nd probiotic serving

Day 14

Breakfast

- 2 scrambled eggs, 4 scrambled egg whites, or 1 scrambled egg plus 2 scrambled egg whites. Top with salsa (optional).
- 1 apple or 1 cup fresh berries
- 1 cup green tea

Lunch

- *Chicken-Vegetable Soup* (page 273)
- 1 cup green tea

Dinner

- Plenty of grilled chicken or fish
- Generous portion of mixed steamed vegetables
- 1 cup green tea

Snacks

- 1 medium pear or other fruit in season
- 2nd probiotic serving of your choice

Day 15

Breakfast

- ½ cup Breakstone's LiveActive cottage cheese
- 1 medium pear, sliced
- 1 cup green tea

Lunch

- *Eggplant Parmesan* (page 274)
- 1 cup green tea

Dinner

- Plenty of broiled lean ground turkey
- *Marinated Vegetable Salad* (page 273)
- 1 cup green tea

Snacks

- 2nd fruit serving of your choice
- 2nd probiotic serving of your choice

Day 16

Breakfast

- *Spanish Omelet* (page 268)
- ½ grapefruit or 1 medium orange
- 1 cup green tea

Lunch
- *Spicy Yogurt Dip and Veggies* (page 272)
- 1 cup green tea

Dinner
- Plenty of roasted turkey breast or turkey tenderloin, steamed carrots and steamed asparagus
- 1 cup green tea

Snacks
- 1 piece fresh fruit
- 6 oz. carton yogurt

Day 17

Breakfast
- *Yogurt Fruitshake* (page 267)
- 1 cup green tea

Lunch
- *Super Salad* (page 269)
- 1 cup green tea

Dinner
- Steamed flounder or sole with lemon pepper
- Steamed broccoli
- 1 cup green tea

Snacks
- 1 medium apple or other fruit in season
- 2nd probiotic serving of your choice

Accelerate Cycle Worksheet

It may help you to plan your meals using the following worksheet. Using the food lists, simply fill in what you will eat each day.

Breakfast

Protein or probiotic serving: _____

Fruit serving: _____

Lunch

Protein or probiotic serving: _____

Cleansing vegetables: _____

Dinner

Protein serving: _____

Cleansing vegetables: _____

Snacks

2nd fruit serving: _____

2nd probiotic serving: _____

Other

Friendly fat serving: _____

Your eating habits may be a lot closer to horrible than healthy right now. That means it's time to hand out pink slips to doughnuts, pizzas, super-burgers, shakes and fries. Your stomach is about to welcome some healthier inhabitants, and I'm going to help you understand what it's like to feel good, and understand the connection between the choices you make and how you feel. For the first 17 days that you follow this diet, you will experience an entirely new energy, and you will see how quickly it can happen and how much better you can feel.

See you (hopefully less of you) in 17 days!

Review
· · · · · · · · · · · · ·

- Cycle 1: Accelerate jump-starts your weight loss.

- This Cycle reduces carb intake slightly and increases protein intake.

- This Cycle clears your body of sugars and toxins to pave the way for weight loss.

- Use my Hunger/Fullness Meter to help you eat just the right amount of food for your body.

- Use this Cycle as a tool to re-ignite weight loss if you ever have a slip and need to get back on track.

THE 17 MINUTE WORKOUT: Get In Two Quickies

Not those kinds of quickies (although you burn calories that way too). What I had in mind are two mini aerobic workouts: 17 minutes in the morning, and 17 minutes in the afternoon or early evening. Science already tells us that exercise boosts your metabolism for a few hours afterward, so just think: you'll nearly double the afterburn if you split it up. Aerobic exercise includes fast walking, jogging, running, exercising on cardio machines and anything that gets your heart pumping for 17 minutes.

The Fiber Factor

Everyone knows about fiber. It is the indigestible part of plant foods our body cannot use for energy. Fiber, which our grandmothers used to call "roughage," travels through our digestive tract creating bulky, soft stools that pass easily. Without adequate fiber, things get stopped up.

The 17 Day Diet is high in fiber on purpose. A growing body of research shows that high-fiber eating helps peel off pounds and banish them for good. Fiber does this mainly by curtailing your food intake. Specifically, fibrous foods provide bulk and stimulate the release of appetite-suppressing hormones. As a result, you feel full while eating a meal, so you're less tempted to overeat.

High-fiber foods also take longer to chew. You may have to chew some foods 42 times before swallowing them. High-fiber foods may even have negative calories, because by the time you have finished chewing them, you have burned up more calories than the food provides. Chewing also makes your meals last longer. That's nice, since it takes about twenty minutes after starting a meal for your body to send signals that it's full. And, when eaten with other nutrients, fiber slows the rate of digestion too, curbing your appetite between meals.

Inhaling fiber-rich foods will have your body running strangely. So make sure you have a good book and some nice soft toilet paper on hand. All of this is good for weight loss, though. The fiber accelerates the time it takes for food to move through your intestinal tract. This means fewer calories are left to be stored as fat.

Attention, everyone reading this: If you eat too much food with a lot of fiber and don't drink enough water, you will have to buy a laxative. Fiber needs water to move through your system, or it will harden up like a block of cement in your colon.

Sally Patton

AGE: **56**

POUNDS LOST: **90**

CURRENT CYCLE: **Activate**

Sally, a contractor for the Wyoming State Department of Health, spends her days managing programs that help citizens use alcohol responsibly, quit smoking, and lead healthier lives. So, at 5 feet 7½ inches and 276 pounds, she felt like a hypocrite teaching folks how to be good to their bodies when she was so dissatisfied with her own health. Part of the problem, she says: "I didn't know I wasn't feeling my best." She had been overweight for the past 30 years. "I didn't know I was fat. I was

generally healthy and active. I just didn't know I was so overweight. I spent 15 years or more on antidepressants, and once I started the 17 Day Diet, I became aware of how far over the edge I was."

She decided to make a change in March 2011, after her best friend tried the program and found success. "What was so nice was that I've been on diets, and this one was simple to understand. The directions are easy, and if you

"If you want to know how fast you can drop 20 pounds, do this plan."

follow it, you get immediate results. It gives you the blueprints for the rest of your life." In the first 17 days, Sally dropped 18 pounds—more than a pound a day. Since she began the program, she has chosen to skip back and forth between Cycles 1 and 2, which helped her lose 90 pounds in just less than a year. Once she hits 100 pounds, she plans to move on to the maintenance phase.

"I've gone from a size 24 to a 12," she says. Now at literally half her former size, she still gravitates to the plus-size section when clothes shopping and has had to retrain herself to look for regular sizes. She's not the only one who has had to adjust. "At 50 pounds, people really noticed. Now, at 90, people don't know who I am. I was at the grocery store and saw this woman we've known for years. She was giving my husband the beady eyes because she thought he was with another woman!"

The journey has been emotional for Sally. She doesn't weigh herself regularly, but when she stepped on the scale at her most recent doctor's appointment, she watched the big metal weight slide down one notch from 200 to the 150 mark. "I cried. It was so awesome. I'm no longer obese."

Sally has noticed all kinds of changes in addition to being leaner: Her skin has become clearer, her cholesterol has dropped back into the healthy range, and she no longer needs to take antacids. In fact, she no longer needs to rely on any of her medications, including her antidepressants. She credits most of these positive changes to the food.

"I get to eat a lot of food. When you're following the diet for the first 17 days, you are so full at the end of the day. You can't eat everything you're supposed to eat." One of the foods that have revolutionized her kitchen is Greek yogurt. "That really satiates me. It's like cheesecake,"

(continued)

Sally Patton *(continued)*

she says, especially when she dresses it up with a dose of Truvia and cinnamon.

"Today I had braised kale with butternut squash and garlic, and tomorrow I won't have carbs," she says, explaining her Cycle 2 routine. One of her favorite breakfasts is oatmeal with raisins and blueberries. For a snack, she likes to keep a resealable plastic bag of kale chips handy, noting that kale is remarkably cheap, even in Wyoming in the middle of winter. All she has to do is spread some kale leaves on a baking sheet, sprinkle them with olive oil and a little salt and bake them. These simple, flavorful foods keep her satisfied and energized. "My tummy feels good. I feel good," she says.

One of the vices she's given up is carbonated soda. "I used to have two Frescas a day. I had one a couple of months ago, and it tasted so horrible and fake I didn't even drink the whole thing." She doesn't crave it anymore, and her stomach has seen smooth sailing ever since. "Now I don't have stomachache or irregularity, and I don't have to take antacids."

Becoming more active has also been a big part of Sally's success. In the beginning, she couldn't even walk the recommended 17 minutes a day, but she gradually built up her endurance. "Now I'm up to six miles a day," she says. Along the way she got a pair of good sneakers, bought her first sports bra, and has even begun experimenting with running. "I never ran in my life. And now every once in a while, I look around, make sure no one's watching, and run." Another healthy habit she has adopted is to keep a pedometer application on her phone so she can log her activity. "I don't push it to pain—I'm not into that. I just like to go."

Perhaps Sally's greatest reward is that she now has the energy to keep up with her young grandkids.

"In my world of being a social worker and victims' advocate and raising kids, I've always taken care of other people. The gift to me has been that this year I've really been able to take care of me."

Her advice:

- Be patient. "The name 17 Day Diet leads you to believe it's a short-term diet, but it takes work."

- Keep your copy handy. "I don't have to read the book every day," Sally says, but she does keep a copy of the book on her Kindle so that she can review the plan when she thinks she has slipped up.

- Don't make her mistake! In the beginning, Sally was drinking eight 16-ounce glasses of water a day. In reality, you should be drinking eight 8-ounce glasses, so be sure to measure at first so you know what that looks like in your standard glasses at home.

4

Cycle 2: Activate

. . . .

If you've been on other diets, you're all too aware of the standard outcome: you cut back on your food and you lose weight . . . at least initially. But then your progress slows to a crawl, before lagging or sometimes stopping altogether. Your body's natural tendency to preserve itself and its fat, at all costs, kicks in. The Activate Cycle corrects this, resetting your metabolism so that your body stays in a fat-burning mode.

This Cycle is easy to follow too: You alternate your Cycle 1: Accelerate days with Cycle 2: Activate days. In other words, you work this Cycle by spending one day on the Activate diet and the next on the Accelerate diet, switching between the two, one day at a time, as you progress toward your goal weight over the next 17 days. Another way to look at it: on odd days you stick to the Activate Cycle; on even days, the Accelerate Cycle.

The approach of alternating Accelerate days with Activate days is based on the scientifically validated mechanism of "alternate-day fasting" (although there is no fasting on this diet in the true sense of the word). In a nutshell, this means alternating low-calorie days with higher-calorie days in order to lose body fat. Scientists at the University of California have led the way in this cutting-edge research, with both human and rat studies. (How many of these furry creatures have lost weight in order to save humanity from obesity during the past 50 years is a mystery to me.)

Publishing much of their research in recent issues of the *American Journal of Clinical Nutrition*, these scientists have unearthed intriguing findings. Alternate-day fasting can:

- Trigger sustained weight loss (no frustrating plateaus). The weight that is lost is mostly fat.

- Activate the "skinny" gene, which tells cells to burn—rather than hold on to—fat.

- Reduce the risk of heart disease by lowering levels of bad cholesterol and triglycerides, decreasing blood pressure and lowering heart rate.

Alternating your food intake is a powerful concept in weight management. Here's a look at what this will be doing for you:

- Stripping away body fat. Your carb intake is still relatively low on this Cycle. When you cut carbs, your muscles give up stored carbohydrates, called muscle glycogen, as energy. In general, when glycogen levels fall, the body increases its ability to burn body fat. Therefore, it makes sense to reduce your carbohydrate intake. When that happens, the body ramps up fat-burning.

- Giving momentum to your metabolism. This potent diet strategy seems to keep the metabolism elevated. It keeps your body guessing, as opposed to letting it get accustomed to one particular way of eating day after day. Just as you need to change things up in workouts for continued progress to avoid plateaus, you mustn't let your body get too comfortable with the foods you

MISTER MD, CAN YOU PLEASE TELL ME ?

Wouldn't it just be easier to prescribe diet pills for weight loss?

Drug companies are always racing to develop new weight-loss drugs, but they haven't had much luck. The Food and Drug Administration has approved only three drugs in the past 30 years for treating obesity, one of which—Redux—was yanked for safety reasons. I don't know what they did with the leftover pills. Maybe they were recycled into something a dieter could use, like exercise bands.

The drugs that remain—Xenical and Meridia—have been moderately successful. But I'm not an advocate of popping pills for every little thing. Pills don't fully address the problem. By prescribing drugs instead of lifestyle changes, doctors ignore the unhealthy habits that have contributed to obesity. One of these diet pills, the "fat blocker" Xenical, the brand name of a drug called orlistat, must be accompanied by a low-calorie diet to reduce your weight by about 5 percent for most. Diets are vital, pills or no pills.

There's an "ick" factor with this particular drug. Fat isn't absorbed, so it has to go somewhere. And orlistat takers find out in a hurry just where. (Keep an extra pair of panties with you, or wear some diapers.)

Yes, some people's obesity is so out of hand that it might be dangerous, and I might prescribe one of these drugs.

About the only advice doctors can give is stop eating sweets, fat, butter, desserts, super-burgers—basically, we want you to avoid anything the least bit tasty. We would make everyone do this if we could. Then we could stop worrying about the obesity epidemic and get back to other things like curing the common cold and filling out insurance forms.

eat. It's all about shocking the metabolism to elicit a positive response.

- Taming your appetite. On the Activate Cycle, you get to eat some starchy carbs. But not just any carbs. You'll eat natural, slow-digesting carbs such as oatmeal, whole grains, brown rice, beans and legumes and sweet potatoes—a whole slew of carbs. Slow carbs take a longer time to reach the blood, which helps you feel full.

- Preventing carb sensitivity. Carbs are beneficial in that they help set up the body hormonally for muscle-toning if you exercise. They spark the release of insulin, which gets protein and carbs into muscles for growth and repair. The downside is that when you take in too many carbs, they can be readily

---

SCIENCE SAYS: Just a Single High-Fat Meal Does Heart Damage

Eating just one single high-fat meal makes your blood pressure go sky high, according to a study by U.S. and Canadian researchers. They fed 30 healthy people a single meal that was either very low-fat (1% of calories) or very high-fat (46% of calories). The high-fat meal was a McDonald's breakfast; the healthier, low-fat meal was cereal and non-fat yogurt. The people were then exposed to stressful situations, such as public speaking, performing mental math and exposure to cold temperatures. Compared to the people given the low-fat meal, those who ate a high-fat meal experienced a greater jump in blood pressure and more stress on their blood vessels. These effects may cause harm to cardiovascular health. So much for the adage "All things in moderation."

Source: *Journal of Nutrition*, April 2007.

converted to body fat and stored. On the Activate Cycle, you're limited to no more than two servings of slow, natural carbs a day. This is the amount most people—especially women—are physiologically capable of tolerating in order to sustain fat metabolism.

Another major difference between the two Cycles is that you get to enjoy a greater variety of lean proteins, including shellfish and beef.

General Guidelines for the Activate Cycle

1. Stay on the Activate Cycle for 17 days. The Activate Cycle consists of alternating between Activate days and Accelerate days.

2. Remove skin from chicken or turkey prior to cooking or purchase skinless poultry.

3. Trim all visible fat from meat.

4. About eggs: You may eat up to two eggs a day. But stick to no more than four yolks per week if your physician has diagnosed you with high cholesterol. Egg whites can be eaten without restriction.

5. Keep gobbling up those fresh fruits and vegetables before they become science-fair-project-worthy in the crisper. For convenience, frozen and canned items are fine, if chosen in moderation. These products should be unsweetened, however.

6. Continue to avoid alcohol and sugar in order to help your body eliminate toxins, improve digestion and burn fat.

7. Don't eat more than two servings daily from the natural starches list.

8. Do not eat your fruit or natural starch serving past 2:00 p.m.

9. Eat slowly and only until full; do not overload your stomach. Use my Hunger/Fullness Meter.

10. Drink eight 8-ounce glasses of pure water a day.

11. Exercise at least 17 minutes a day.

Take More Off: The Activate Cycle Food List

On the Activate Cycle, you'll be adding new foods to those you ate on the Accelerate Cycle. These additional foods are listed below.

Proteins

Add in the following foods:

Shellfish

Clams	Mussels	Scallops
Crab	Oysters	Shrimp

Lean Cuts of Meat* (The leanest cuts are those from the part of the animal that gets the most exercise. Therefore, cuts from the round, chuck, shank and flank are the best.)

Beef round tip	Pork boneless loin roast
Beef top loin	Pork sirloin chops
Beef top sirloin	Pork tenderloin
Eye of round	Pork top or center loin chops
Flank steak	Top round
Lamb shanks	Top sirloin steak
Lamb sirloin roast	Veal cutlet
Lean ground beef	

*Lean cuts tend to be a little tougher. You can tenderize lean cuts by marinating in fat-free liquids like fruit juice, wine, fat-free salad dressings or fat-free broth.

Natural Starches

Grains (½ cup = 1 serving)

Amaranth

Barley, pearled

Brown rice

Bulgur

Coucous

Cream of wheat

Grits

Longer grain rice such as Basmati

Millet

Oat bran

Old-fashioned oatmeal

Quinoa

Legumes (½ cup = 1 serving)

Black beans

Black-eyed peas

Butter beans

Garbanzo beans (chickpeas)

Great Northern beans

Kidney beans

Lentils

Lima beans, baby

Navy beans

Peas

Pinto beans

Soy beans

Split peas

Starchy Vegetables

Breadfruit (1 cup = 1 serving)

Corn (½ cup = 1 serving)

Potato (1 medium = 1 serving)

Sweet potato (1 medium = 1 serving)

Taro (½ cup = 1 serving)

Winter squashes (acorn, spaghetti, butternut, etc.) (1 cup = 1 serving)

Yam (1 medium = 1 serving)

Cleansing Vegetables

(Same foods as Accelerate Cycle)

Low-Sugar Fruits

(Same foods as Accelerate Cycle)

Probiotics

(Same foods as Accelerate Cycle)

Friendly Fats

(Same foods as Accelerate Cycle)

Condiments

Condiments and seasonings are allowed in moderation: salsa, low-carb marinara sauce, lite soy sauce, low-carb ketchup, fat-free sour cream, low-fat, low-sodium broth, Truvia (a non-caloric sweetener made from natural ingredients), sugar-free jams and jellies, vegetable cooking spray, fat-free cheeses (e.g. Parmesan), fat-free salad dressing, salt, pepper, vinegar, mustard, herbs and spices.

Meal Planning Made Easy

On Activate days, you eat:

- Liberal amounts of protein and cleansing vegetables.
- Two daily servings of natural starches (carbohydrates).
- Two low-sugar fruit servings.
- Two servings of probiotic foods.
- One daily serving of friendly fat.

Here's a typical day on the Activate Cycle:

Breakfast
- ½ cup hot whole grain cereal or 2 eggs or 4 egg whites, prepared without oil; 1 *Dr. Mike's Power Cookie*; or one probiotic serving
- 1 fruit serving
- 1 cup green tea

Lunch

- Liberal amounts of protein in the form of fish, shellfish, meat, chicken or eggs, or vegetables plus 1 probiotic serving

- 1 serving natural starch

- Unlimited amounts of cleansing vegetables

- 1 cup green tea

Dinner

- Liberal amounts of protein in the form of fish, shellfish, meat, or chicken or turkey

- Unlimited amounts of cleansing vegetables

- 1 cup green tea

Snacks

- 2nd fruit serving

- 2nd probiotic serving

Additional

- 1 friendly fat serving (1 to 2 tablespoons of olive oil or flaxseed oil to use on salads or vegetables, or for cooking)

Remember: Follow one day of the Activate Cycle with a menu from the Accelerate Cycle, and alternate accordingly for a total of 17 days.

17 Sample Menus

Here are examples of how to create your daily meals during the Activate Cycle. You may follow these exactly or create your own menus based on the above guidelines. Recipes are in Chapter 14.

Wake-up drink

Every morning, as soon as you rise, drink one 8-ounce cup of hot water. Squeeze half a lemon into the cup; the lemon stimulates your digestive juices. Your goal is to drink at least six to seven more glasses of water by the end of the day. The rate at which you burn calories drops if you're dehydrated. And if you're dehydrated, your body doesn't absorb nutrients properly.

Day 1

Breakfast

- *Dr. Mike's Power Cookie* (page 266)
- 1 fresh peach, sliced
- 1 cup green tea

Lunch

- Chicken salad: baked or grilled chicken breast (diced), loose-leaf lettuce, 1 sliced tomato, assorted salad veggies, 2 tablespoons olive oil mixed with 4 tablespoons balsamic vinegar
- ½ cup brown rice
- 6 oz. sugar-free fruit flavored yogurt

Dinner

- Grilled salmon
- Steamed veggies

Snacks

- *Yogurt Fruitshake* (page 267)

Day 2

- Accelerate Cycle menu

Day 3

Breakfast

- 2 scrambled egg whites
- ½ grapefruit, or other fresh fruit of your choice
- 1 cup green tea

Lunch

- *Chicken-Vegetable Soup* (page 273) or grilled chicken breast and plenty of steamed veggies
- 1 medium baked potato with 1 tablespoon fat-free sour cream ("Medium" means it fits in the cup of your hand.)
- 6 oz. sugar-free fruit-flavored yogurt
- 1 cup green tea

Dinner

- Sirloin steak, grilled
- Tossed salad with 1 tablespoon olive oil and 2 tablespoons balsamic vinegar
- 1 cup green tea

Snacks

- 1 cup fresh raspberries (or other in-season fruit) with 1 cup sugar-free fruit-flavored yogurt
- Mediterranean spread: ½ cup garbanzo beans (pureed and mixed with 1 tablespoon olive oil) and served on cucumber slices

Day 4

- Accelerate Cycle menu

Day 5

Breakfast

- ½ cup oatmeal or grits, cooked
- 4 egg whites, scrambled
- 1 fresh peach, sliced
- 1 cup green tea

Lunch

- Shrimp salad: cooked shrimp, 3 tablespoons chopped onion, generous bed of lettuce leaves, 1 tomato (large) and 1 tablespoon olive oil
- 1 baked sweet potato, medium
- 1 cup green tea

Dinner

- Pork sirloin chops, broiled or grilled
- Steamed veggies
- 1 cup green tea

Snacks

- 1 cup blueberries with 6 oz. sugar-free fruit-flavored yogurt
- 6 oz. sugar-free fruit-flavored yogurt or 1 cup kefir

Day 6

- Accelerate Cycle menu

Day 7

Breakfast

- 2 eggs, scrambled without oil

- 1 baked potato, diced, seasoned and browned in a small frying pan that has been coated with vegetable cooking spray
- 1 orange or other fresh fruit in season
- 1 cup green tea

Lunch
- *Turkey Black Bean Chili* (page 276)
- Large tossed salad with 1 tablespoon olive oil mixed with 2 tablespoons vinegar and seasoning
- 1 cup green tea

Dinner
- Extra lean hamburger patty, broiled
- Sliced fresh tomatoes, drizzled with fat-free salad dressing
- Green beans or other veggie, steamed
- 1 cup green tea

Snacks
- *Kefir Smoothie* (page 267)
- 6 oz. sugar-free fruit-flavored yogurt

Day 8
- Accelerate Cycle menu

Day 9

Breakfast
- ½ cup Breakstone's LiveActive cottage cheese
- 1 medium pear, sliced
- 1 cup green tea

Lunch

- Grilled chicken breast
- ½ cup pinto beans
- ½ cup cooked corn
- 1 cup green tea

Dinner

- Grilled salmon
- Steamed broccoli
- Sliced fresh tomato drizzled with 1 tablespoon olive or flaxseed oil mixed with vinegar and seasonings
- 1 cup green tea

Snacks

- 1 medium apple
- 6 oz. sugar-free fruit-flavored yogurt

Day 10

- Accelerate Cycle menu

Day 11

Breakfast

- *Kefir Smoothie* (page 267)
- 1 cup green tea

Lunch

- Plenty of broiled hamburger
- 1 medium baked potato
- ½ cup peas

Dinner

- Plenty of roasted turkey breast

- Steamed asparagus

- Large tossed salad with 1 tablespoon olive oil mixed with 2 tablespoons vinegar and seasonings

Snacks

- 1 medium orange

- 6 oz. sugar-free fruit-flavored yogurt

Day 12

- Accelerate Cycle menu

Day 13

Breakfast

- *Dr. Mike's Power Cookie* (page 266)

- 1 medium peach, sliced

- 1 cup green tea

Lunch

- *Low-Carb Primavera Delight* (page 276)

- 1 cup green tea

Dinner

- Plenty of London broil

- Large tossed salad with 1 tablespoon olive oil mixed with 2 tablespoons vinegar and seasonings

- 1 cup green tea

Snacks

- *Yogurt Fruitshake* (page 267)
- 2nd probiotic serving of your choice

Day 14

- Accelerate Cycle menu

Day 15

Breakfast

- 1 cup lean granola (such as Kashi Go Lean) mixed with 6 oz. sugar-free fruit-flavored yogurt (*Note:* 1 cup of lean granola gives you your 2 servings of natural starch for the day.)
- 1 cup green tea

Lunch

- Fruit salad: ½ cup Breakstone's LiveActive cottage cheese with diced fruit (½ cup diced strawberries and ½ cup diced peach) served on a generous bed of lettuce
- 1 cup green tea

Dinner

- Grilled pork chops
- Steamed or boiled cabbage
- Large tossed salad with 1 tablespoon olive oil mixed with 2 tablespoons vinegar and seasonings
- 1 cup green tea

Snacks

- 1 medium apple or pear
- 2nd probiotic serving of your choice

Day 16

- Accelerate Cycle menu

Day 17

Breakfast

- 2 cooked eggs (scrambled, poached, etc., without oil)
- 1 cup fresh berries
- 1 cup green tea

Lunch

- Grilled chicken breast
- 1 medium sweet potato or ½ cup mashed butternut squash
- ½ cup cooked corn
- 1 cup green tea

  (*Note:* The servings of sweet potato and/or squash plus corn give you your 2 servings of natural starch for the day.)

Dinner

- Grilled or boiled shrimp
- Steamed green beans
- Large tossed salad with 1 tablespoon olive oil mixed with 2 tablespoons vinegar and seasonings
- 1 cup green tea

Snacks

- 1 medium orange or nectarine
- 2nd probiotic serving of your choice

LEAN 17:   Lost in Spice—17 Ways to Make Veggies and Other Foods Taste Great

When you're on a diet, you've got to get creative. Here are some suggestions to get the most flavor from your food, without using added fat or sugar.

1. Basil. Basil adds loads of flavor to tomato-based dishes. It's also great with poultry.

2. Broth. Use low-sodium, low-fat chicken and beef broth to sauté meats and cook flavorful rice without adding oil.

3. Cayenne pepper. Just a pinch livens up chili, spaghetti squash and salad dressings. Consuming cayenne may help suppress your appetite. When a group of men and women took 900 milligrams of cayenne pepper a half hour before meals, they felt fuller and reduced their calorie and fat intake, according to a study appearing in the June 2005 issue of the *International Journal of Obesity*.

4. Chives. Add 1 part chopped chives to 3 parts spinach and boil or steam for 3 minutes.

5. Cinnamon. Sprinkle this sweet spice in oatmeal, hot cereals or coffee. A 2003 study published in *Diabetes Care* reported that as little as one gram of cinnamon reduced blood glucose and cholesterol levels in type 2 diabetics.

6. Dill. Known mostly as a pickle herb, dill is delicious on fish, carrots and salads. For an easy dip, mix it into plain yogurt and serve with cucumber slices.

7. Garlic. Stir it into mashed potatoes or salad dressing.

8. Horseradish. Ditch the gravy and go for horseradish to enliven meat. Or puree it into Breakstone's LiveActive cottage cheese, along with some garlic and pepper, for a healthy vegetable dip or potato topping.

9. Italian seasonings (generally a combination of oregano, rosemary, savory, marjoram, basil and thyme). Sprinkle it on chicken, spaghetti squash, vegetables and tomatoes.

10. Lemon. Squeeze fresh juice on salads, vegetables and fish. Grate the rind to create the zest (flavorful outer rind). This gives a tang to poultry, vegetables and salads.

11. Mint. You can't beat fresh mint from your garden, but dried mint is tasty, too. Good in tea, with fruit, and in plain yogurt.

12. Mustard. Dijon mustard adds zip to many dishes, from turkey burgers to roasted potatoes.

13. Rosemary. The fragrant, needle-like leaves of this woody herb are especially good with lamb and seafood, and in any dish with beans, tomatoes, onions, potatoes or cauliflower.

14. Sage. This Mediterranean herb is especially good in tomato-based dishes, beans, tuna, chicken or turkey.

15. Tarragon. This wonderful seasoning makes salads and chicken taste delicious. For your salad dressings, try tarragon vinegar mixed with olive oil or flaxseed oil.

16. Thyme. A member of the mint family, thyme is great on carrots, cauliflower, Brussels sprouts and beef.

17. Vinegar. Try cider vinegar on cooked spinach, herbed or raspberry vinegar on salad greens, rice vinegar on chicken salad and malt vinegar on broiled fish.

SCIENCE SAYS: The Truth about High-Fructose Corn Syrup

Maybe you've seen the pro-high-fructose corn syrup (HFCS) ads running on television. First, the ads say that HFCS is no worse than sugar. Well, that's like saying cigars are no worse than cigarettes. Second, the ads say HFCS is natural because it's made from corn. C'mon, so is ethanol, and I'm not slurping that down either.

Let me set the record straight. HFCS is a cheap gooey sweetener used in soft drinks, meats, cheeses and dozens of other foods. Recent studies have raised many health concerns about the syrup. HFCS:

- Is linked to obesity. A steadily rising consumption of HFCS parallels closely with a rise in obesity. Also, HFCS very quickly turns into body fat, in some cases never even yielding energy for the body to use. One can of soda a day (the equivalent of 10 teaspoons of sugar) can lead to a 10-pound fat gain in just one year.

- Increases triglycerides, a recognized risk factor for heart disease. Also, people with elevated triglycerides overproduce a chemical component called the superoxide free radical. This molecular pickpocket can damage a variety of cell structures, including DNA, and is thought to promote aging.

Raises blood pressure, another risk for heart disease.

Causes the body to over-produce insulin. High insulin is one of the earliest signs of type 2 diabetes.

Is linked to the risk of nonalcoholic fatty liver disease. This is the most prevalent form of progressive liver disease in the United States. In this disease, the liver gets inflamed and scarred. At that point, it can cause cirrhosis or liver cancer and ultimately liver failure.

Was shown in a small study to make pancreatic cancer cells proliferate. Scientists put these cancer cells in lab dishes and fed them glucose and fructose (fructose is a sugar in HFCS). The cells gobbled up the fructose and left the glucose alone.

Should you be consuming less HFCS? Yes! Limit your intake of all added sweeteners, including HFCS, fructose, sucrose (table sugar), glucose and corn syrup. In fact, as a doctor, I'd also suggest you skip soft drinks and fruit juices altogether.

Sources: *World Journal of Gastroenterology*, 2010; and *Cancer Research*, 2010.

Activate Cycle Worksheet

It may help you to plan your meals using the following worksheet. Using the food lists, simply fill in what you will eat each day.

Activate Day

Breakfast

Protein or probiotic serving: _____

Natural starch serving: _____

Fruit serving: _____

Lunch

Protein or probiotic serving: _____

Natural starch serving: _____

Cleansing vegetables: _____

Dinner

Protein serving: _____

Cleansing vegetables: _____

Snacks

2nd fruit serving: _____

2nd probiotic serving: _____

Other

Friendly fat serving: _____

Accelerate Days

Breakfast

Protein or probiotic serving: _____

Fruit serving: _____

Lunch

Protein or probiotic serving: _____

Cleansing vegetables: _____

Dinner

Protein serving: _____

Cleansing vegetables: _____

Snacks

2nd fruit serving: _____

2nd probiotic serving: _____

Other

Friendly fat serving: _____

Review

- Cycle 2: Activate is based on "alternate day fasting," in which you alternate lower-calorie days with slightly higher-calorie days. Here you alternate Activate days with Accelerate days.

- Alternating your diet days charges up your metabolism and helps prevent dreaded weight-loss plateaus.

- Additional foods such as natural carbs are re-introduced to your diet on this Cycle.

By the time you finish the Activate Cycle, provided you've done it without cheating, you'll have enough of a weight loss that your clothes are starting to get too baggy and loose for you. Don't lose focus now, because you're doing great.

Simmie Sinow

AGE: **61**

POUNDS LOST: **91**

CURRENT CYCLE: **Arrive**

Simmie began the 17 Day Diet in February 2011. In the first 17 days alone, she dropped 11.8 pounds, and over the course of the year, she has become almost 100 pounds slimmer. "I didn't want it to be all about the numbers. I reached my clothing size goal one day before my one-year anniversary of being on the diet," she says proudly. Thanks to the 17 Day Diet, Simmie has deflated from a size 24 to a 12.

But she couldn't do it alone. One of her biggest cheerleaders is the 86-year-old woman for whom she works as a caregiver in San Diego, California. "My client has been totally supportive of my weight-loss journey. She says, 'Keep at it; if you don't lose weight this week, you will next week.' But I've never gone a week without losing weight."

In fact, Simmie's health has seen a complete overhaul. She sleeps better, she feels she is more mentally focused and her digestive health has completely turned around. "Going

"I've lost 91 pounds and six clothing sizes in just less than a year!"

into this, I had IBS, and food went right through me." Eating the wholesome, unprocessed foods on the 17 Day Diet has brought her intestines under control, she says. "I don't even take my GERD medication once a month. That has been just wonderful. I would wake up in the middle of the night with heartburn that was just killing me, and I don't have that anymore."

Friends and family have really taken notice. Her roommate's son, a personal trainer, has praised her success and is now giving her exercise advice and strength workouts to try. "My roommate and I went out for a long walk this morning with our two dogs. Back when I started, I wouldn't have been able to make it halfway. Now I can go there and back and I'm ready for more," Simmie says. And her favorite moment so far? "I saw my ex-husband at a brunch last week, and he e-mailed me afterward and said, 'You look fantastic.' He's a Marine, so for him to say that, that was something else."

Earlier this year, Simmie became the moderator of one of the 17 Day Diet fan groups on Facebook.com. Since then, the group has shot up from 1,800 members to 4,200, and Simmie does her best to keep up with words of encouragement and advice. She and a team of 19 other 17 Day Dieters have even created their own "17 Day Diet Test Kitchen" where they create recipes for each cycle of the plan. One of her cotesters came up with a flourless pancake recipe, muffin bites and some other really delicious recipes. As for Simmie, "I get really creative with smoothies," she says. Her favorite is to take kefir, a scoop of vanilla whey protein powder and orange sugar-free Jell-o powder. She adds some flaxseed or sticks it in the freezer to thicken it up, and then it tastes just like a Creamsicle, she says. For breakfast, she'll add fresh blueberries to the kefir and sometimes spinach—which you don't taste, Simmie says,

(continued)

Simmie Sinnow *(continued)*

but it does turn the smoothie green. Her friends call it the "Green Monster Smoothie."

Being able to eat good food is an essential part of staying on the plan for Simmie. She's lucky that many meals she already loves fit right in—like chicken Parmesan. But for the most part, she relies on substitutions and recreated recipes. For example, birthdays can be hard, but she found a solution. "There's always cake, and I love the frosting on cake. In our test kitchen we *just* came up with a recipe for that." Now, when she decorates desserts, she uses frosting with a cream cheese base, ditching the sugar for vanilla whey powder and Truvia. You can get the whole recipe (and many others) at 17ddgal.blogspot.com.

"Give it 51 days for the first 3 Cycles and see what a difference it makes. It will change your life. It has changed mine incredibly."

Advice to other 17 Day Dieters?

- Check with your doctor. Simmie's doctor was thrilled with her weight loss and was able to offer personalized modifications based on Simmie's health history that she wouldn't have had if she hadn't brought it up at her appointment.

- To avoid constipation, be sure to drink enough water and eat high-fiber foods. For quick relief, taking 250 milligrams of magnesium twice a day helps for Simmie. But everyone is different, so be sure to check with your doctor.

5

Cycle 3: Achieve

· · · · · · · · · · · · · ·

You have been on the 17 Day Diet for 34 days now. Yes, I'm counting. We should be seeing less of you, since French fries and candy bars are no longer homesteading on your hips. You're looking great, fitting beautifully into clothes and, I hope, pleased with your progress.

Now is the time to start adding new food choices, including things like pasta. Pasta is not the archenemy of the human body, by the way. But portions the size of national monuments are. Every food group is represented on Cycle 3, and there's still an emphasis on non-starchy vegetables and lean protein. Now you can enjoy some alcohol, unless you're going to drive, you're under 21, you're pregnant or you're defusing a bomb or working in a nuclear power plant.

On this Cycle, you'll eat moderately, and continue to do some form of exercise that works your cardiovascular system, only I want you to step up the duration of your workouts.

There are fewer food rules on this Cycle. But yes, food eaten over the sink or stove, or otherwise while you're standing up, still counts in your daily intake.

CHECKUP: Your Progress

☐ I have lost a pleasing number of pounds.

☐ My clothes fit better.

☐ I have dropped a dress size.

☐ I have more energy.

☐ People have noticed my weight loss and complimented me.

☐ I feel more motivated to treat my body with respect.

☐ I feel less hungry.

☐ I am sleeping better.

☐ My skin looks better.

☐ My elimination has improved.

☐ My stomach is flatter.

☐ I feel lighter.

☐ I have fewer cravings.

☐ My mood is better.

I call this Cycle Achieve because one of its chief purposes is to help you achieve good lifetime eating habits, such as portion control, regular mealtimes and the inclusion of healthy foods.

Some of you may have already reached your goal weight, particularly if you had just 10 or 15 pounds to take off. Congratulations. You may collect a Get-Out-of-the-Achieve-Cycle-Free Card and go right to Cycle 4.

For the rest of you, before we get started on Achieve Cycle 3, let's talk about what positive changes you've begun to enjoy. Look at my check-up on this page. Mark any changes that apply. Make a copy of the check-list and stick it on your fridge so that the next time you feel like nosing around in the freezer for that 20-inch pizza that you forgot to throw out, the list will stop you in your tracks.

The Speed of Weight Loss on Cycle 3

So far, you have been dropping weight at the speed of light, or just about. On Cycle 3, expect your weight loss to slow down a bit. I tell you this so that when you get on the scales, you won't be disappointed, blow your diet big-time, and vow not to start up again until next January.

The goal of this Cycle is to establish healthy eating habits and produce steady, manageable weight loss. So just relax and enjoy the addition of whole grain breads and pasta, additional fruits and vegetables, fats and snacks and alcohol in moderation (one alcoholic drink a day).

Okay, now that I've told you your weight loss may slow down a bit over the next 17 days, let me tell you how to speed it up on Cycle 3. You can do this in three ways:

1. **Ramp up your aerobic exercise.**

   Aerobic exercise, such as walking, jogging, biking or aerobics classes, is the best way to burn fat and speed up weight loss. So if you've been doing it at least 17 minutes a day, it's time to add even more minutes. Aim to do 45 to 60 minutes of aerobic exercise most days of the week.

2. **Continue not to eat carbs after 2:00 p.m.**

   During Cycles 1 and 2, I recommend not eating carbs after 2:00 p.m. If you did a good job of replenishing your muscle and liver glycogen throughout the day—which is what carbs do—then any excess carbs in the later afternoon and at night—a time when you're typically least active—will be readily converted to fat. On Cycle 3, you're allowed to have carbs at dinner. But if you want to spur weight loss, continue avoiding carbs after 2:00 p.m.

3. **Pass on the alcohol.**

   I know I just gave you the thumbs-up for alcohol on Cycle 3. But please know that alcohol can throw a complete monkey wrench into weight loss. Alcohol strains your liver, which responds by slowing down on functions like fat-burning. Alcohol is also dehydrating and will cause water-weight pounds to register on the scale. If you want bigger losses on this Cycle, pass up the alcohol option.

Achieve Cycle Guidelines

1. Stay on the Achieve Cycle for 17 days.

2. Because you'll be eating more food, it's time to control your protein portions. Rather than eat protein liberally as in the 2 previous Cycles, keep your portions of fish, poultry and meat smaller—about the size of an average kitchen sponge. In fact, you can use that sponge to sop up any remnants of fat that might have dripped off the protein.

3. Remove skin from chicken and turkey prior to cooking or purchase skinless poultry.

4. Trim all visible fat from meat.

5. You may eat up to two eggs a day. But stick to no more than four yolks per week if your physician has diagnosed you with high cholesterol. Egg whites can be eaten without restriction.

6. Enjoy fresh vegetables and fruits as much as possible. For convenience, frozen and canned items are fine, if chosen in moderation. Canned and frozen fruits should be unsweetened.

7. You may have one alcoholic drink daily: 5 oz. wine; 12 oz. beer; or 1½ oz. hard liquor if you wish. Attention, everyone reading this: Notice I said, "one." If you go to a party, have one drink and spend the rest of the night drinking nonalcoholic, calorie-free drinks such as flavored seltzer. (This will help you avoid embarrassing work-party karaoke moments.) Please remember that alcohol has a dehydrating effect and can interfere with fat-burning and weight loss. One drink per day, however, has a positive effect on cholesterol levels. Accumulating evidence suggests that moderate drinking may lower the risk of heart attacks.

MISTER MD, CAN YOU PLEASE TELL ME ?

When's the best time of day to exercise?

The short answer: the best time of day to work out is the time that works for you.

Luckily, some scientists have been working on this. But scientists are like judges on *American Idol*. They don't agree on anything, and so their findings always conflict.

As for morning workouts, people burn 10 percent more fat calories with early-morning workouts, one study shows. Bodybuilders, who are not scientists, swear by exercising in the morning before breakfast. They claim it is the best time to shed flab. Supposedly, after a night of sleeping, your carb stores are lower, so your body is forced to go to your fat stores for fuel. But what do bodybuilders know? They only leave the gym for bodybuilding contests and more protein powder.

Most doctors will agree with me on the following: Do not try pre-breakfast exercise under the following conditions: (1) if you are a diabetic or suffer from low blood sugar, because you could become dizzy or nauseous; or (2) if you are not much of a dawn's-early-light person and a morning workout sounds about as appealing as watching reruns of *Are You Smarter Than a 5th Grader?*

As for evening workouts, a recent study by a group of Italian scientists found that women who walked in the evening burned more fat than women who walked in the morning. It's not clear why, though.

Again, there's no bad time to exercise, except for maybe right now, when I'm hoping you're reading this chapter.

8. Don't eat more than two servings daily from the natural starches list.

9. Don't worry about eating all the food you're allowed each day. If you forget your second dairy or carb serving, or are too full to eat it, that's okay.

10. Eat slowly and only until full; do not overload your stomach. Use my Hunger/Fullness Meter as a gauge to keep you from stuffing yourself.

11. Begin to increase your weekly aerobic exercise. Exercise at least 150 to 300 minutes per week, depending on your physical condition (five 30-minute sessions or five 60-minute sessions).

Achieve Cycle Expanded Food List

Where indicated, add foods to your diet, in addition to those you ate on the first 2 Cycles.

Proteins

Fish and shellfish (from Accelerate and Activate lists)

Lean meats (from Accelerate and Activate lists)

Poultry (from Accelerate and Activate lists, including eggs and egg whites)

Additional poultry:

Canadian bacon

Cornish hen

Quail

Pheasant

Reduced-fat turkey bacon or sausage or lunch meat

Natural Starches

Breads (1 slice = 1 serving)

Cracked wheat bread

Fiber-enriched bread

Gluten-free bread

Multi-grain bread

Oat bran bread

Pumpernickel

Rye bread

Sugar-free bread

Whole grain bagel (½ = 1 serving)

Whole wheat pita bread, 1 pocket

Whole wheat tortilla (10")

SCIENCE SAYS: If You Have to Drink Alcohol on Your Diet, Drink Red Wine

Okay, here we are back on the alcohol issue. There is some intriguing research I want to share with you about one of my favorite food groups, red wine. I mentioned earlier that red wine contains a heart-protective compound called resveratrol, which does everything but fly to the moon. Apparently, resveratrol can also reduce the number of fat cells in a person's body, and scientists think it may one day be used to treat or prevent obesity. Several years ago, researchers at the University of Ulm in Germany took a strain of human fat cell precursors, called preadipocytes. In the body, these are "baby" cells that develop into mature fat cells.

In this cell-based study, they found that resveratrol inhibited the pre-fat cells from increasing and prevented them from converting into mature fat cells. Also, resveratrol hindered fat storage.

This makes sense when you think about French women. French women are skinny, even though they eat a high-fat diet and drink lots of wine. In fact, according to the most recent statistics, French women also have Europe's lowest average Body Mass Index—the measure of weight that takes into account someone's height.

Scientists think the resveratrol in red wine is a fat-burner—and why the French can eat gobs of fat and still stay thin.

Source: *American Journal of Clinical Nutrition,* 2010.

High-Fiber Cereals (1 cup = 1 serving, except where indicated)

All-Bran

All-Bran Bran Buds

All-Bran Extra

Fiber One

Gluten-free cold cereals

Low-sugar granola (½ cup = 1 serving)

Pasta (½ cup = 1 serving)

Gluten-free pasta	Vegetable-based pasta
High-fiber pasta	Whole wheat pasta
Udon noodles	

Vegetables—Unlimited

All cleansing vegetables	Nopales (edible cactus)
Alfalfa	Pea pods
Broccoli sprouts	Radishes
Chiles	Rhubarb
Cilantro	Rutabaga
Fennel	Summer squash
Grape leaves	Swiss chard
Jicama	Yellow wax beans
Kelp and other edible seaweeds	Zucchini
Kohlrabi	*Virtually any vegetable*

Fruits—2 servings daily*

Apricots	Mango
Bananas	Papaya
Cherries	Pineapple
Currants	Pomegranate
Figs	Tangelo
Kiwi	Tangerine
Kumquats	*Virtually any fresh fruit*
Guava	

*Serving = 1 piece fresh or 1 cup chopped fresh fruit

Note: If you are watching your sugar intake, stick to lower-sugar fruits. These include apples, berries (all varieties), cherries, grapefruit, oranges, peaches, pears, and plums.

Probiotics, Dairy and Dairy Substitutes—1 to 2 servings daily

Note: Some people don't like dairy foods, or can't digest them properly. If you're one of them, try dairy substitutes instead (see below). Try to eat at least one serving daily from this list while on the Achieve Cycle.

Probiotic foods from Accelerate and Activate Cycles

Low-calorie cheeses (brie, camembert, fontina, low-fat cheddar, edam, feta, goat, limburger, and part-skim mozzarella) (2 ounces = 1 serving)

Low-fat cottage cheese (½ cup = 1 serving)

Low-fat milk, including skim (1 cup = 1 serving)

Low-fat ricotta cheese (½ cup = 1 serving)

Dairy substitutes: Sugar-free rice, almond or soy milk (1 cup = 1 serving)

Friendly Fats—1 to 2 tablespoons daily, except where indicated

Avocado (¼ fruit = 1 serving)

Canola oil (1 tablespoon = 1 serving)

Walnut oil (1 tablespoon = 1 serving)

Light mayonnaise (2 tablespoons = 1 serving)

Mayonnaise (1 tablespoon = 1 serving)

Nuts or seeds, unoiled (2 tablespoons = 1 serving)

Reduced-calorie margarines (2 tablespoons = 1 serving)

Reduced-fat salad dressings (2 tablespoons = 1 serving)

Salad dressings (1 tablespoon = 1 serving)

Trans-free margarines (1 tablespoon = 1 serving)

Optional Snacks

These snacks are all under 100 calories. Plus, they're filling and fun to eat.

Babybell low-fat cheese—2 disks

Frozen fruit bar

Fudgsicle, 100-calorie bar

Granola bar, reduced sugar and fat

Microwave popcorn, light (4 cups)

Skinny Cow ice cream sandwich

Sugar-free pudding cup

String cheese—1 stick

Meal Planning Made Easy

Each day, for the next 17 days, you'll eat:

- Controlled portions of protein from an expanded list.
- Liberal amounts of vegetables from an expanded list.
- 2 servings of natural starches from an expanded list.
- 2 servings of fruit from an expanded list.
- 1 to 2 servings of probiotics, low-fat dairy or dairy substitutes.
- 1 serving of fat from an expanded list.
- Optional snacks.
- Optional daily serving of alcohol.

Here is a typical day on the Achieve Cycle:

Breakfast

- ½ cup hot whole grain cereal; or 2 eggs or 4 egg whites,

prepared without oil; 1 *Dr. Mike's Power Cookie*; or 1 probiotic serving

- 1 fruit serving

Lunch
- Controlled portions of protein in the form of fish, shellfish, meat, chicken or eggs; or vegetables + 1 probiotic, dairy or dairy substitute serving

---

SCIENCE SAYS: Liposuction Has Health Benefits

Thinking about getting liposuction? Talk to your doctor. Liposuction, like all procedures, has risks. But liposuction has been found to help reverse type 2 diabetes and reduce cholesterol.

As I mentioned earlier, obesity makes your body's cells resistant to insulin. The result is that sugar can't enter your cells, and your blood-sugar level rises. Liposuction seems to reverse that process. In a study at Brooklyn's Downstate Medical Center, a surgeon removed an average of 12 pounds of fat from seven young women with type 2 diabetes. After the procedure, their cells lost their insulin resistance, and their blood-sugar levels dropped. The findings are intriguing. This was a small study, so it will be interesting to see if future studies into liposuction improve insulin resistance too.

The other benefit of liposuction is this: Removing just 6 pounds of fat can lower your cholesterol level dramatically. That's the conclusion of University of Salzburg researchers. They think sucking off just small amounts of fat shifts a patient's metabolism for the better.

Although I prefer you help your health the old-fashioned way—diet, exercise, determination, willpower and dedication—these studies hold promise.

- 1 serving natural starch
- Unlimited amounts of vegetables

Dinner

- Controlled portions of protein in the form of fish, shellfish, meat, chicken or turkey
- Unlimited amounts of vegetables

Snacks

- 2nd fruit serving; or
- 2nd probiotic, dairy or dairy substitute serving; or
- Food from optional snack list

Additional

- 1 serving (1 to 2 tablespoons of friendly fat to use on salads, vegetables, or for cooking)

17 Sample Menus

Here are examples of how to build menus while on the Achieve Cycle. You can follow these exactly or create your own.

Wake-up drink

Every morning, as soon as you rise, drink one 8-ounce cup of hot water. Squeeze half a lemon into the cup; the lemon stimulates your digestive juices. Your goal is to drink at least six to seven more glasses of water by the end of the day. The rate at which you burn calories drops if you're dehydrated. And if you're dehydrated, your body doesn't absorb nutrients properly.

Day 1

Breakfast
- 1 slice whole wheat toast
- 1 poached, soft-boiled or hard-boiled egg
- ½ grapefruit
- 1 cup green tea

Lunch
- Chicken Caesar salad: grilled chicken breast, cut in pieces; 2 cups Romaine lettuce; other desired salad veggies; 2 tablespoons light Caesar dressing
- 1 slice whole- wheat toast
- 1 serving fresh fruit
- 1 cup green tea

Dinner
- Roasted pork tenderloin
- 1–2 cups tossed mixed salad with 2 tablespoons fat-free dressing
- 1 cup green tea

Snacks
- 1 probiotic, dairy or dairy substitute serving
- 1 frozen fruit bar

Day 2

Breakfast
- 1 cup cereal, high-fiber (e.g. Bran Buds or Fiber One)
- 1 cup (8 oz.) skim, 1% or soy milk or other dairy substitute

- 1 cup fresh berries
- 1 cup green tea

Lunch

- Pita sandwich: 1 whole wheat pita filled with chopped lettuce and tomato; 2 tablespoons crumbled fat-free feta cheese; 1 table-spoon Italian salad dressing
- 10 baby carrots
- 1 cup green tea

Dinner

- Barbecued chicken: boneless, skinless breast with barbecue sauce; grill or bake until done
- Steamed vegetables such as asparagus, wax beans, broccoli or cauliflower
- 1 cup green tea

Snacks

- 2nd fruit serving
- 1 Skinny Cow ice cream sandwich

Day 3

Breakfast

- 1 cup plain yogurt
- 1 sliced banana
- 1 slice cracked wheat toast
- Jam, 1 tablespoon (to mix with yogurt or on toast)
- 1 cup green tea

Lunch

- Peel-and-eat shrimp (boiled or steamed)
- ¼ cup cocktail sauce
- ½ cup reduced-fat coleslaw (you can prepare a low-fat version by mixing a bag of coleslaw with reduced-fat coleslaw dressing)
- 1 medium baked sweet potato
- 1 cup green tea

Dinner

- Grilled or broiled salmon
- Green beans, steamed, or other veggie
- 1 cup green tea

Snacks

- 2nd fruit serving
- 2nd probiotic, dairy or dairy substitute serving

Day 4

Breakfast

- *Dr. Mike's Power Cookie* (page 266)
- 1 cup (8 oz.) skim, 1% or soy milk or other dairy substitute
- 1 cup fresh berries
- 1 cup green tea

Lunch

- Lean ground beef (browned) mixed with low-carb marinara sauce and served over ½ cup whole wheat or gluten-free pasta
- 1–2 cups tossed mixed salad with 2 tablespoons reduced-fat dressing
- 1 cup green tea

Dinner

- *Chicken-Vegetable Soup* (page 273)
- 1 cup green tea

Snacks

- 2nd fruit serving
- 2nd probiotic, dairy or dairy substitute serving
- 1 Skinny Cow ice cream sandwich

Day 5

Breakfast

- 2 scrambled eggs
- 2 slices reduced-fat turkey bacon
- 1 cup fresh berries
- 1 cup green tea

Lunch

- Tuna sandwich: tuna mixed with 1 tablespoon mayonnaise, chopped celery and onion, served between two slices of whole grain bread
- 1 fresh pear
- 1 cup green tea

Dinner

- *Low-Carb Primavera Delight* (page 276)
- 1 cup green tea

Snacks

- Probiotic, dairy or dairy substitute serving
- One 100-calorie Fudgsicle

Day 6

Breakfast

- 1 cup sugar-free fruit flavored yogurt
- ½ cup lean granola
- 1 piece fresh fruit (e.g. 1 peach, ¼ cantaloupe, ½ grapefruit or 1 orange)
- 1 cup green tea

Lunch

- Tomato stuffed with crab salad: Mix lump crab meat with 1 tablespoon light mayonnaise and 2 tablespoons chopped celery and serve on a generous bed of lettuce.
- Medium baked potato with 1 tablespoon fat-free sour cream; or ½ cup brown or Basmati rice
- 1 medium apple
- 1 cup green tea

Dinner

- Roast beef, eye of round
- Zucchini, sautéed with 1 tablespoon olive oil and Italian spices
- 1 cup green tea

Snacks

- 2nd probiotic, dairy or dairy substitute serving
- 1 frozen fruit bar

Day 7

Breakfast

- ½ cup low-fat or fat-free cottage cheese
- 1 cup pineapple chunks, fresh or canned in their own juice
- 1 cup green tea

Lunch

- Grilled cheese sandwich: Place 2 light cheese singles and 2 slices tomato on 2 slices whole wheat bread and cook in pan sprayed lightly with vegetable spray until toasty and cooked throughout.

- 1 cup baby carrots or other chopped fresh veggies

- 1 cup green tea

Dinner

- Baked chicken thighs, skinless

- Steamed vegetables

- 1–2 cups tossed mixed salad with 2 tablespoons reduced-fat dressing

- 1 cup green tea

Day 8

Breakfast

- *Dr. Mike's Power Cookie* (page 266)

- 1 banana, sliced

- 1 cup non-fat or acidophilus milk

- 1 cup green tea

Lunch

- *Turkey Black Bean Chili* (page 276)

- 1 serving fresh fruit

- 1 cup green tea

Dinner

- Grilled salmon

- 1–2 cups tossed mixed salad with 2 tablespoons fat-free dressing

- 1 cup green tea

Snacks

- 1 probiotic, dairy or dairy substitute serving
- 1 frozen fruit bar

Day 9

Breakfast

- ½ cup lean granola
- 6 oz. sugar-free fruit-flavored yogurt
- 1 cup fresh berries
- 1 cup green tea

Lunch

- *Super Salad*
- 1 cup green tea

Dinner

- Sirloin steak
- 1 medium baked potato, topped with 1 tablespoon fat-free sour cream (optional)
- Steamed vegetables such as asparagus, wax beans, broccoli or cauliflower
- 1 cup green tea

Snacks

- 2nd fruit
- 1 Skinny Cow ice cream sandwich

Day 10

Breakfast

- ½ cup cooked oatmeal
- ½ grapefruit
- 1 cup green tea

Lunch

- *Nicoise Salad* (page 269)
- 1 cup green tea

Dinner

- Baked turkey breast
- 1 medium baked sweet potato
- Green beans, steamed, or other veggie
- 1 cup green tea

Snacks

- 2nd fruit serving
- 2nd probiotic, dairy or dairy substitute serving

Day 11

Breakfast

- *Spanish Omelet* (page 268)
- 1 medium apple or pear
- 1 cup green tea

Lunch

- Lean ground beef (browned) mixed with low-carb marinara sauce and served over ½ cup whole wheat or gluten-free pasta

- 1–2 cups tossed mixed salad with 2 tablespoons reduced-fat dressing
- 1 cup green tea

Dinner
- *Sesame Fish* (page 274)
- Steamed green beans
- ½ cup acorn or butternut squash
- 1 cup green tea

Snacks
- 2nd fruit serving
- 2nd probiotic, dairy or dairy substitute serving
- 1 Skinny Cow ice cream sandwich

Day 12

Breakfast
- 4 scrambled egg whites
- 1 slice Canadian bacon
- 1 cup melon balls
- 1 cup green tea

Lunch
- Chicken sandwich: grilled or baked chicken mixed with 1 tablespoon mayonnaise, chopped celery and onion, served between 2 slices whole grain bread
- 1 fresh pear, or other fruit in season
- 1 cup green tea

Dinner

- 2 broiled lamb chops
- Steamed broccoli or cauliflower
- Cooked carrots
- 1 cup green tea

Snacks

- Probiotic, dairy or dairy substitute serving
- One 100-calorie Fudgsicle

Day 13

Breakfast

- 1 cup sugar-free fruit-flavored yogurt
- 1 piece fresh fruit (e.g. 1 peach, ¼ cantaloupe, ½ grapefruit or 1 orange)
- 1 cup green tea

Lunch

- Turkey sandwich: reduced-fat turkey, 1 slice reduced-fat Swiss cheese, mustard, lettuce, slice of tomato—between 2 slices rye bread
- 1 medium apple
- 1 cup green tea

Dinner

- Baked chicken breast
- Zucchini, sautéed with 1 tablespoon olive oil and Italian spices
- 1 cup green tea

Snacks

- 2nd probiotic, dairy or dairy substitute serving
- 1 frozen fruit bar
- 1 cup green tea

Day 14

Breakfast

- 2 scrambled eggs
- 1 slice whole grain toast
- 1 cup pineapple chunks, fresh or canned in their own juice
- 1 cup green tea

Lunch

- *Lettuce Wraps* (page 272)
- Light fries: Bake frozen potato or sweet potato french fries, keeping to portion recommended on the package.
- 1 cup green tea

Dinner

- Broiled turkey burger
- 1–2 cups tossed mixed salad with 2 tablespoons reduced-fat dressing
- 1 cup green tea

Day 15

Breakfast

- *Yogurt Smoothie*
- 1 slice whole wheat toast
- 1 cup green tea

Lunch

- Chicken Caesar salad: grilled chicken breast, cut in pieces; 2 cups Romaine lettuce; other desired salad veggies; 2 tablespoons light Caesar dressing
- 1 serving fresh fruit
- 1 cup green tea

Dinner

- Roasted pork tenderloin
- 1 medium sweet potato or ½ cup mashed butternut squash
- 1 cup green tea

Snacks

- 1 probiotic, dairy or dairy substitute serving
- 1 frozen fruit bar

Day 16

Breakfast

- 1 cup cereal, high-fiber (e.g. Bran Buds or Fiber One)
- 1 cup (8 oz.) skim, acidophilus, 1% or soy milk or other dairy substitute
- 1 banana, sliced
- 1 cup green tea

Lunch

- *Taco Salad* (page 271)
- 1 cup green tea

Dinner

- *Oven Barbecued Chicken* (page 275)

- Steamed vegetables such as asparagus, wax beans, broccoli or cauliflower
- 1 cup green tea

Snacks
- 2nd fruit serving
- 1 Skinny Cow ice cream sandwich

Day 17

Breakfast
- 1 cup plain yogurt
- 1 cup fresh berries
- Jam, 1 tablespoon (to mix with yogurt)
- 1 cup green tea

Lunch
- Peel-and-eat shrimp (boiled or steamed)
- ¼ cup cocktail sauce
- ½ cup corn
- 1 cup green tea

Dinner
- Steak
- 1 medium baked potato with 1 tablespoon sour cream
- 1–2 cups tossed mixed salad with 1 tablespoon oil mixed with 2 tablespoons vinegar
- 1 cup green tea

Snacks

- 2nd fruit serving

- 2nd probiotic, dairy or dairy substitute serving

- 1 fat-free pudding cup

Achieve Cycle Worksheet

It may help you to plan your meals using the following worksheet. Using the food lists, simply fill in what you will eat each day.

Breakfast
Protein or probiotic or low-fat dairy serving: _____

Starch serving: _____

Fruit serving: _____

Lunch
Protein: _____

Starch serving: _____

Vegetables: _____

Dinner
Protein serving: _____

Vegetables: _____

Snacks
2nd fruit serving: _____

2nd probiotic or low-fat dairy serving: _____

Optional snack: _____

Other
Friendly fat serving: _____

SCIENCE SAYS: Snooze, You Lose (Weight)

Researchers are learning more about how critical sleep is to slimming down. Adequate sleep keeps important appetite and weight-loss hormones in balance so that you stay satisfied by what you eat. Lack of sleep throws off levels of these hormones. Also, people are less likely to make healthy choices when they're tired.

Doctors have a long history of missing sleep, which may explain why many doctors are fat. Being sleep-deprived goes back to our internship days when we had to stay up for 30 hours straight sometimes. Once I nodded off for a moment and almost strangled myself with my stethoscope.

If you don't have enough time to sleep at night, try to schedule at least a short power nap during the day. Napping can contribute to weight loss, according to a study in the *American Journal of Physiology, Endocrinology, and Metabolism*. (That should be great news unless you have a newborn in the house, or you're apt to get fired for sleeping on the job.)

Anyway, the study looked at hormone levels in 41 men and women who were part of a seven-day sleep-deprivation experiment. Those allowed to nap for two hours following a night without any sleep showed a significant drop in cortisol, a hormone related to high levels of stress, and weight gain around the belly.

So forget counting calories and start counting sheep.

If You Have More Weight to Lose

At the end of Cycle 3, if you have additional weight to lose, you have several options:

- Return to Accelerate for 17 days, continue to Activate for 17 days, and follow with Achieve for 17 days; or

MISTER MD, CAN YOU PLEASE TELL ME ?

Why can't I drink diet sodas on the 17 Day Diet?

Well, you can. Just don't tell me about it.

Diet soda sure seems like a dieter's dream: You can swill down as much as you want, and none of it will glom onto your thighs, right? Wrong. This bubbly beverage has a sneaky MO to make you put on pounds. Here's how: Diet soda is flavored with artificial sweeteners, which can be many times sweeter than regular sugar. That super-sweet taste can instantly trigger your natural desire for high-calorie, sugary foods. The more you drink, the worse those cravings can be, prompting you to reach for real sweets. Have diet soft drinks in moderation, but concentrate more on drinking water, sparkling water, or seltzer, all of which keep cravings on an even keel without sparking a junk-food binge.

- Return to Activate for 17 days, and follow with Achieve for 17 days; or

- Continue on with Achieve until you reach your goal weight.

Suggestion: If you are very close to your goal weight at the end of your first Achieve Cycle, it's best to return to the Accelerate Cycle for up to 17 days to reach your goal more quickly.

As we wrap up this Cycle, think for a moment about how good it feels to slim down. Replacing those lost pounds should be newfound feelings of self-control, increased health and fitness, loose clothing, continual compliments, improved physical appearance, excitement and an overall boost of pride. I know it hasn't been easy. But the accomplishment of losing weight will bring you true satisfaction—something a Happy Meal could never do.

Review

- Cycle 3: Achieve is a more moderate, liberalized food plan that allows a wide range of healthy foods, eaten in proper portions for continued weight loss.

- Weight loss may slow down during Cycle 3, but you can speed it up by (1) increasing your aerobic exercise; (2) not eating carbohydrates of any type past 2 p.m.; and (3) avoiding optional alcohol.

- The purpose of Cycle 3 is to help you achieve good eating habits.

Maha Nasrallah

AGE: **30**

POUNDS LOST: **39**

CURRENT CYCLE: **Arrive**

. . . .

Maha, an architect and freelance photographer in Abu Dhabi, United Arab Emirates, first heard about the 17 Day Diet while watching *Dr. Phil*. Sick of being overweight, she decided that she wanted to slim down before her 30th birthday that coming November. She convinced her sister May to try the program with her, and they started it together in June 2011. Cycle 1 was very challenging for the pair. Maha recalls, "By day five, I was dying to have a sandwich." Instead of the carb-filled meals the sisters were accustomed to having, they subsisted on the prescribed yogurt for breakfast, tuna salad for lunch, and skinless, boneless chicken breasts for dinner—plus snacks of fruit, veggies, and an additional yogurt depending on the day. It was a dramatic change from their old eating habits, especially when it came to snacks. "We were really used to mindless eating, whether biscuits, chocolate or anything," Maha says. Dining out also became hard. One of her biggest challenges during the first two cycles was that her social life suffered since she usually spent her time with friends eating out at restaurants. "I'd order green tea and watch my friends eat," she lamented. "It was not very easy. But what got me through it was that I saw fast results."

Maha lost about 11 pounds in the first 17 days, and her sister lost roughly the same. They stuck with the program and by October 2011, Maha had dropped from a size 14 down to a 6! Best of all, she successfully met her goal right before the big 3-0. "It was awesome

"I gave up my old wardrobe."

turning 30. I was healthy, fit, and slim—and finally a runner!"

Now she is nearly 40 pounds lighter and half her size. "People don't recognize me," she says. Acquaintances sometimes ask Maha if she has had surgery and she's happy to reply that no, she just exercised and ate right.

"Now, to be honest, the first two months I would run to the mirror and check to make sure I wasn't fat. And every time I look at my reflection, I get surprised. I hardly recognize the person staring back at me. Not that I mind it!"

The 17 Day Diet has changed many things for Maha—her skin glows now, and she admits that she just feels better when she eats healthfully. After getting used to fresh, wholesome foods, she finds that fast food is much too salty and greasy to her now.

But the best part of dropping all those extra pounds is that shopping for clothes has never been better! "I go and try on clothes just for fun," she reports, explaining that her style has done a complete 180. Now she isn't afraid to wear more figure-hugging outfits, and she owns a lot more dresses. She actually gave up her entire old wardrobe—except for one pair of "fat pants." "Whenever I forget my achievement, I wear them and feel better," she says.

Though active before, Maha really ramped up her exercise program once she committed to the 17 Day Diet. For a while, she worked with a personal trainer who helped show her how to get the right mix of cardio and strength routines. "He has become one of my best friends," she says, "but I train on my own now." These days she runs for exercise, and she recently completed her first half-marathon. Though she still follows the 17 Day Diet's fourth Cycle and relies on the strategic cheating to keep herself on track, she also looks to her favorite magazines, like

(continued)

Maha Nasrallah *(continued)*

Women's Health and their e-newsletters, to keep her primed with the latest diet and exercise information.

"I indulge from time to time, especially sweets," Maha says, but she says she'll never go back to her old eating habits and sedentary lifestyle. "No, I can't go back. It's what got me in trouble. If I overeat during a meal, I try to watch it for the next one. Now weekends are a bit hard to control, so I try to behave during the week." One of her favorite fast fixes is creamy frozen yogurt whenever an ice cream craving hits. This low-carb solution works great on Cycles 3 and 4.

She continues to stick the program because it's simple and the results are real. "The rules are very clear. You know what to do, and you just need to have a strong will to keep doing it."

Her advice:

- "Hang in there. I know it's tough and I know there are times when you just feel like giving up. And it's OK to feel that way—to just want to wake up and be slim and healthy. But if you just stick to it, you will cross the finish line. It will be sooo worth the sacrifice."

- Once you have made it through all four cycles once, if you have more weight to lose or need to get back on track after indulging a little too much, don't feel restricted to going back to Cycle 1—pick a pattern that feels doable. "When I was desperate to lose 5 pounds, I did Cycle 1. I barely survived three days," she laughs. "So Cycle 3 came to the rescue."

Cycle 4:
Arrive

. . . .

You made it! Applause, everyone!

You started the 17 Day Diet, and you decided you'd do it for just 17 days. That worked wonders, so then you committed to another 17 days, and another. You felt so good about yourself and proud of your achievement, that you decided to go right to your goal. By stringing those 17 day Cycles together, you reached that goal.

You fought the battle of the bulge and won! Now it's time to keep the bulge at bay, but how? With what I call the Arrive Cycle, because you've *arrived* at your goal weight. This is a huge, important accomplishment, something many people fail to do. Now, the important thing is that you stay at this weight.

At this point in the book, I have to be really, really honest, and talk about a big unmentionable thing, something no one wants to acknowledge.

You will always be on some kind of diet.

You will not be able to return to your former eating habits and keep the weight off, because those very habits—like eating way too many super-sized fast-food meals and being inactive—created the weight in the first place. So you've always got to diet, if you want to maintain this weight loss. Maintenance plans, in the dieting vernacular, really mean nothing more than following another diet.

Whaddaya mean, I've got to diet forever?

Yes, it's true, you've always got to watch your weight. Sorry. Keeping weight off is a bear, a big, hungry, growling one. Once a dieter, always a dieter.

Got that? Okay, so at least let's have some fun doing it.

What I propose as a "keep-it-off strategy" is weekends off.

Let's face it: weekends have never been good for diets. You get a promotion on Friday, so you eat. Or you snuggle up to watch a video on Friday or Saturday, and you eat. Or you go out to a party, and you eat. The problem is, from 6:00 p.m. on Friday until bedtime on Sunday, your life changes. Your schedule is looser, allowing for more snacking. Then there are the social commitments. Dinners out, birthday shindigs, Sunday brunch—they can do you in. It seems like you need thick layers of duct tape on your mouth to prevent pig-outs.

Taking weekends off allows you to splurge a bit, making it easier to get back on track on Monday. Most people can be pretty disciplined Monday through Thursday, choosing meals carefully, getting in some exercise, and seeing decent results on the scale. The Arrive Cycle capitalizes on these normal rhythms of life and builds a *livable* maintenance plan around them.

In a nutshell, here's how you keep weight off: Stay strict during the week and then enjoy yourself more over the weekend. Most people do this to lose weight. I advise that you do it to keep weight off.

I'm giving you the best diet present you can have. You still eat a calorie-controlled diet during the week, then on weekends, have what you like. You take off plenty of pounds, and you keep the weight off because you never get bored using my weekend principle.

The Arrive Cycle is metabolically strategic, too. You can control your weight efficiently because you're shocking your metabolism back into action. Why? Because you're following five days of controlled eating, followed by two days of increased calories. By adding calories to your meals—with hamburgers, bread, ice cream, wine, cheesecake, you name it—you're speeding up your metabolism. Then, when your metabolism is roaring like a furnace, you get back to your diet on Monday, burning calories faster than ever. Basically, the Arrive Cycle keeps your metabolism guessing, so it never has a chance to go into hibernation. Since your metabolism is now well trained due to better eating habits and digestive health, a few cheat treats on the weekend will not have an adverse effect.

The Arrive Cycle is not a free-for-all. You're allowed some of your favorite foods in moderation. For example: Friday night, a restaurant meal with a cocktail or two at your favorite restaurant. Saturday, a slice or two of pizza for lunch or dinner, plus one dessert. Sunday, a breakfast of pancakes with maple syrup.

A good rule of thumb to follow while stabilizing your weight is to enjoy no more than one to three "favorite meals" each weekend.

I call this "strategic cheating."

I must add a warning: if the only time you aren't putting things in your mouth is while you're asleep, you may have an eating disorder, or a history of one. If so, this way of eating is not for you. But, 99 percent of dieters who follow the 17 Day Diet are ready and motivated to live the Arrive Cycle, and I'll give you some super-easy strategies to make sure strategic cheating on weekends doesn't turn into pigging out during the week.

Breathe a sigh of relief. Life is about to get normal, with you locked in at a normal, healthy, beautiful weight.

Start the Arrive Cycle

The Arrive Cycle is unique in that it helps you keep your weight off, while letting you enjoy yourself and eat freely from your favorite foods on weekends.

Basically, the Arrive Cycle works like this:

- Monday breakfast through Friday lunch: Enjoy meal plans from one of your favorite Cycles: Accelerate, Activate or Achieve.

- Friday dinner through Sunday dinner: Enjoy your favorite foods and meals in moderation over the weekend.

- Enjoy no more than one to three favorite meals over the weekend. Do not binge. Eat slowly and enjoy your food.

- If desired, enjoy alcoholic drinks in moderation over the weekend (1 to 2 daily): 1½ oz. hard liquor, 5 oz. wine or 12 oz. beer.

- You may include soups in your daily menus, as long as they are broth-based. Avoid soups made with milk or cream. Having soup prior to a meal will help curb your appetite and help you feel full.

- As one of your fruit servings, you may substitute fruit juice (unsweetened), but no more than ¾ cup per serving.

- Feel free to enjoy 1 cup of vegetable juice as a snack.

- Continue to use condiments in moderation. Choose non-fat, low-calorie seasonings, such as reduced-fat dressings, spices, herbs, lemon or lime juice, vinegar and hot sauce.

- Exercise on weekends, as well as weekdays.

- Each Monday, I'd like you to renew your commitment to yourself and to your new incredible body. Do this, and you'll control your eating week by week, with a strategy that'll guarantee success.

The Arrive Cycle Lifestyle

Let me give you an example of how this Cycle works in real life. Mary lost 30 pounds on the 17 Day Diet. To keep those pounds off, she follows the Accelerate Cycle Monday through Friday. For the weekends, she plans meals in which she will enjoy her favorite foods. Whatever she wants the most, she lets herself have on those designated weekend days. Planning is key; it is far better than spontaneous splurges.

"It was important for me to know that I had these little treats coming," Mary says. "But it was even more important to know that I would get right back on the 17 Day Diet on Monday, and I always did."

Here's a look at Mary's typical week:

Monday

Breakfast
- 6 oz. plain low-fat yogurt, mixed with 1 cup berries or other fruit (chopped)
- 1 cup green tea

Lunch
- A large salad with lots of different cleansing vegetables and some flaxseed dressing
- 1 medium apple
- 1 cup green tea

Dinner
- Plenty of grilled or baked salmon
- Liberal amounts of cleansing vegetables, steamed or raw
- 1 cup green tea

Snacks
- 6 oz. sugar-free fruit-flavored yogurt or 1 cup plain low-fat yogurt
- Baby carrots, raw, for nibbling

Tuesday

Breakfast

- 2 scrambled eggs
- 1 medium pear or other fruit in season
- 1 cup green tea

Lunch

- Broiled hamburger
- Sliced or stewed tomatoes
- 1 cup green tea

Dinner

- A stir-fry of vegetables (broccoli, onions, julienne carrots, red pepper, etc.) and chicken strips with 1 tablespoon olive oil
- 1 cup green tea

Snacks

- 1 cup fresh berries with 6 oz. yogurt
- 1 bowl of low-fat, low-sodium chicken broth with miso (low-sodium)

Wednesday

Breakfast

- ½ cup Breakstone's LiveActive cottage cheese
- 1 medium orange
- 1 cup green tea

Lunch

- Tuna on a generous bed of salad greens with fat-free salad dressing
- 1 medium apple
- 1 cup green tea

Dinner

- Grilled chicken breast
- Steamed asparagus
- Side salad drizzled with 1 tablespoon olive or flaxseed oil, mixed with 2 tablespoons balsamic vinegar and seasonings
- 1 cup green tea

Snacks

- 6 oz. yogurt
- Raw, cut-up veggies, for nibbling

Thursday

Breakfast

- 2 hard-boiled or poached eggs
- ½ grapefruit or other fresh fruit in season
- 1 cup green tea

Lunch

- Baked turkey breast
- Tomatoes, sliced or stewed, drizzled with 1 tablespoon flaxseed oil
- 6 oz. yogurt
- 1 cup green tea

Dinner

- Grilled salmon
- Steamed green beans
- 1 cup green tea

Snacks

- 1 medium orange
- 1 cup acidophilus milk or 6 oz. yogurt

Friday

Breakfast
- *Kefir Smoothie* (page 267)
- 1 cup green tea

Lunch
- Grilled chicken tossed with reduced-fat salad dressing, served over a generous bed of lettuce
- 1 cup green tea

Dinner out with Friends
- Vegetable lasagna
- Tossed salad with blue cheese dressing
- Wine, two 5 oz. glasses
- Tiramisu, 1 serving

Snacks
- 1 medium apple
- 6 oz. yogurt

Saturday

Breakfast
- 2 scrambled eggs
- ½ grapefruit
- 1 cup green tea

Lunch
- Grilled salmon on a generous bed of lettuce with reduced-fat salad dressing
- 1 cup green tea

Dinner at a Steakhouse

- Grilled ribeye steak
- Caesar side salad with dressing
- 1 medium baked sweet potato
- Two 5 oz. glasses of wine

Snacks

- 1 cup fresh berries
- 1 cup acidophilus milk or 6 oz. yogurt

Sunday

Brunch

- Blueberry waffles with 2 tablespoons syrup
- Turkey sausage, 2 patties
- 1 cup orange juice

Dinner

- Grilled chicken breast
- Steamed broccoli
- 1 cup green tea

Snacks

- 6 oz. sugar-free fruit-flavored yogurt or 1 cup plain low-fat yogurt
- Baby carrots, raw, for nibbling

Analyze Mary's week. Note that it exemplifies a reasonable, moderate way of eating. She sticks to her diet during the week, but gives herself a little leeway on the weekends. "Yes, I'll treat myself. I love Italian food and good wine, and I get to enjoy it on the weekends. Come Monday, I just go right back to fruits and vegetables and chicken and fish," she says.

Mary planned her three favorite meals for the weekend. The rest of the time, she ate prudently, following the Accelerate Cycle. Mary walks briskly most days of the week and always on the weekends. There's no way she's going to regain any weight. Sometimes, she even loses weight.

The Arrive Cycle is about being healthier and smarter about your selections and not pigging out. If you want to have some fried chicken on the weekends, you can do it. You're compensating by having healthier foods through the week. All is not lost. You don't really have to eliminate those foods. It's more about moderation and how to balance those foods in your diet with healthier meals.

Never fool yourself into thinking you can go back to your old eating habits. It is important to hang onto your new habits and eat wisely. As Mary did, all you have to do is follow your favorite Cycle, basically five days a week, then take the weekends off. And make sure you exercise.

Arrive Cycle Strategies

I want to give you a bagful of Arrive Cycle tricks to keep you going. In my experience with patients, the following factors are essential for keeping the bulge at bay.

Observe the Five-Pound Stop Signal

On the Arrive Cycle, weigh yourself on the weekends. Anytime you see the scale register three to five pounds over your weight goal, go right back on your favorite Cycle, Accelerate, Activate or Achieve, on Monday. Note: You'll always get back to your normal weight faster by resuming the Accelerate Cycle. If, for some reason, you've gained a great deal of weight (perhaps by being on vacation), your solution is to start the 17 Day Diet from the beginning and progress through all Cycles.

I know you're saying "ugh" right now, but hear me out. Researchers looked at thousands of people on the National Weight Control Registry who had lost 60 pounds or more and kept it off. The scientists found that 44 percent of the subjects weighed themselves daily. You don't have to go that far, but I do recommend weekend weighing. The number you see in the morning may keep you from going overboard. One of the bedrocks of permanent weight loss is accountability, so I urge you to check the scale on both days of the weekend.

Oftentimes, busy lives take over after the "diet," and people do not notice even large gains in weight. It's much easier to lose three pounds than 20. Plus, studies show that people who stop weighing themselves regain weight. Don't let that happen to you!

Be a Breakfast Lover

On most diets, people starve themselves in the morning so they can eat more for lunch and dinner. This doesn't work. Eat breakfast. Heck, anytime someone tells you to eat, you really should listen!

You really do need to eat breakfast. You say you're not that hungry in the morning? Okay, but eat anyway, because research shows that eating first thing will make you feel more satisfied throughout the entire day, and you'll consume fewer calories, all told. Even on weekends. What's more, I've personally found that most people who skip breakfast become ravenous by 10:30 that morning and often find themselves eating whatever is on hand, even if it's really fattening junk food.

Get on Good Terms with Salad

Have a salad when you dine out or eat at home. According to a study at Penn State University, starting dinner with a large salad may help lower the number of calories you'll consume at that meal. What kind of salad are we talking about? I think you know the answer. No, not a few leaves of romaine underneath a mountain of cheese and croutons. I'm talking about salad veggies topped with one tablespoon of light dressing.

Make Healthier Substitutes

Try to eat certain reduced-fat, reduced-sugar foods. These include:

- Mustard instead of mayo on sandwiches
- Skim milk instead of the whole stuff
- Fake butter sprays
- Salsa for dipping
- Reduced-sugar ketchup or steak sauce
- Fat-free, sugar-free ice cream and frozen treats
- Fat-free sour cream on baked potatoes instead of butter and sour cream
- Fat-free or reduced-calorie salad dressings
- Grilled chicken or turkey sandwiches instead of burgers at fast-food joints

Every little bit helps.

Exercise Portion Control

What's the major dietary blunder of the last 10 years? Ginormous portions of rice and pasta and boulder-size potatoes and yams. Large portions and rich food in restaurants are a major source of extra calories for Americans, a fact not likely to change soon. (More on this in Chapter 9.) It's important to recognize this and to continue to choose well when out, and control portion sizes. Pay attention to portion sizes, and don't reach for seconds.

Move It, Keep It Off

I said you could eat more food on the weekend, but I'm also saying you should burn off more of that food. Think about it: the weekend is when you have more time, usually, to exercise—so take advantage of your free time. Get in at least an hour of intense, heart-pumping exercise on Saturday and Sunday. If you do this, it will be a cinch to keep your weight off. Exercise is one thing that really keeps you thin and fit.

Find ways to sneak in "lifestyle activity" too, especially on weekends. Yard work is a great example. What I see now are people sitting on riding lawnmowers with grass-catching capabilities—the kind that was used by farmers to clear the "back 40." Now people are using it to mow a patch of grass the size of a bath mat. Lawn mowing is great exercise, but only if you push the mower. It burns 387 calories an hour!

Here's what other weekend chores burn per hour:

LEAN 17: 17 Weekend Chores That Incinerate Calories (per hour)	
1. Watering lawn and garden by hand	102
2. Cleaning, dusting	176
3. Moderate housework	246
4. Carpentry, general	246
5. Plumbing	246
6. Gardening	281
7. Bagging grass	281
8. Raking lawn	303
9. Weeding or planting a garden	317
10. Painting	317
11. Cleaning gutters	352
12. Ax chopping, slow	362
13. Remodeling	387
14. Shoveling snow	422
15. Moving heavy objects (like helping your kid move to college)	528
16. Farming, baling hay, cleaning barn	563
17. Trimming trees	633

Avoid Overboard Syndrome

Never binge. Translated: No pig-outs. No stuffing your face until it grows to the size of a basketball. Get your eating under control. Decide that this way of eating is going to change.

Make lists of trouble foods that might make you binge. Deep down, you know what these foods are, so it's best to not include them in your weekend treat meals.

Plan your week's meals in advance, so you're programming your brain and stomach to expect food. It will help you stop eating out of habit.

Stick to one of the Cycles during the week; enjoy your favorite foods on the weekends. But use your head. Go ahead and include pizza in your nutrition plan—just choose a single slice, not the whole pie! Maintain that consistency, and you'll be thin for life.

No More Guilt Trips

On the Arrive Cycle, there's no need to struggle with the dieter's mentality that one bad or good deed will either break or make your weight-loss efforts. You have permission to indulge—as long as it's planned and doesn't spin out of control into weekdays. You're in control; food is not in control of you. Remembering this will help you bounce back into wise eating on Monday.

And if you ever falter? Pick yourself up and get back on the program. None of us are perfect, so there's nothing gained by beating ourselves up and returning to unhealthy, even destructive, patterns of behavior. The healthiest option is to laugh it off and get back to business as soon as you can. Don't worry about doing it to perfection. Just do it.

Stay Focused

I often repeat the phrase "If you always do what you always did, you'll always get what you always got." This mantra will help you remember that if you revert to old habits, then the pounds will pack right back on. Remind yourself of how great you look. Keep pictures of your new self at home, at work, even in your wallet. Look at them whenever you're coming up with excuses not to exercise or considering a trip to the vending machine. Eventually you'll stop and think each time you're about to undermine your diet. In the meantime, the pictures will help you to hesitate. Also, list reasons you never want to get fat again and put them in random places next to your slim pictures. Also, wear tight clothing (it should fit well now) so you stop eating when you feel fat. That's a little trick one of my patients taught me.

The truth about the Arrive Cycle is that it involves more than following a diet. It's about making a permanent change in behavior. This is a lifestyle change, a new way of living. You can now manage a lifetime of good nutrition, enjoy food, and keep fat from creeping back on.

THE 17 MINUTE WORKOUT: Be a Human Pretzel and Keep Weight Off

The slow stretches and meditations of yoga don't burn calories like a run on the treadmill. But a new study suggests yoga might help people *keep weight off*, especially if you're in middle age. Middle-age people of normal weight generally put on pounds over 10 years, but those who did yoga gained less weight than those who didn't practice yoga.

The link between yoga and weight control has nothing to do with burning calories, since with yoga you don't actually torch much fat. Researchers believe that yoga helps keep people more in tune with their bodies and eating habits and aware of bad habits, such as eating because of stress, boredom or depression. Also, people who practice yoga tend to avoid junk food and overeating because they want to respect their bodies.

Source: *Alternative Therapies in Health and Medicine*

LEAN 17:   "Healthy" Foods That Will Make You Fat

Some foods with healthy reputations are actually worse for your weight than you might think. Take a look.

Food	Fattening Factor
1. Dried fruit	Cup for cup, dried fruit has tons more calories than the fresh kind because it has been dehydrated and is much denser. Fresh grapes, for example, have 60 calories per cup, while raisins have 460.
2. Granola	It's loaded with good-for-you nuts and oats, but loaded with oil and sugar for more flavor. One bowl racks up around 500 calories. Try low-fat granola instead.
3. Bran muffins	Most bran muffins are basically just a round slice of cake. One muffin can weigh in at about 20 grams of fat, 420 calories and 34 grams of sugar.
4. Bagel	Many bagels weigh four to five ounces. At 80 calories per ounce, that's a 320- to 400-calorie hunk of bread. Stick to small, whole wheat bagels.
5. Half-and-half	It seems harmless; after all, you put so little in your coffee or tea. But a few spoonfuls per cup of Joe two or three times a day quickly turns into 200 or more calories, plus the same amount of fat as a big pat of butter.
6. Flavored coffees	Drinks at coffeehouses will sabotage your diet faster than you can say Frappuccino. Some of these items top out at 700 calories a serving.
7. Bottled teas	Most store-bought brands are souped up with sugar or honey. Oh, and one bottle can contain two or more servings, bringing the calorie count to almost 200, similar to a can of soda.

Food	Fattening Factor
8. Rice cakes	These light snacks are fat-free and low in calories, but they're also completely lacking in fiber or protein—ingredients that can tame your hunger. That means downing two or three won't do anything but add more calories to your daily total and leave you craving something with substance.
9. Juice	Juice is basically sugar and calories. A 16-ounce bottle of orange juice or apple juice has 55 grams of carbohydrates, the equivalent of five slices of bread. And most of that is sugar: a whopping 12 spoonfuls of it.
10. Fat-free frozen dessert	The label might say it's as low as 60 calories for a small cup, but lab tests on these frozen delights say otherwise: around 270 calories is more like it.
11. Reduced-fat cookies	Three of these will give you 150 calories. But get this: three regular chocolate-chip cookies are 160 . . . just 10 measly calories more.
12. Energy bars	The average candy bar has 250 calories; so does the average energy bar. Energy bars are candy bars incognito, disguised by a few added vitamins (which you're better off getting from fruit). Personally, I'd rather have a Snickers.
13. Energy drinks	The labels say they contain various herbs, minerals and the amino acid taurine, specially designed to boost your energy. But if you look at the ingredients, they're mostly caffeine and sugar, making them hardly more than high-priced soft drinks.
14. Diet drinks	The artificial sweeteners they contain make it harder for people to regulate their calorie intake. Sweet tastes tell the brain a lot of calories are about to be consumed. When that doesn't happen, you eat more to compensate.

(continued)

Food	Fattening Factor
15. Taco salad	One of these can weigh in at more than 900 calories (that's if you eat the hard-to-resist shell). Try my recipe for taco salad instead.
16. Trail mix	Just three little tablespoons of this snack packs around 140 calories. Most people gobble down much more than that, making this a very high-calorie snack.
17. A bag of popcorn at the movies	A medium bag weighs in at 900 calories—and that's without the butter.

THE 17 MINUTE WORKOUT: 17 Ways to Burn More Calories without Jogging

Activity	Effort Expended
1. Run errands	Walking briskly while lugging dry cleaning or groceries can burn about 120 calories in 30 minutes.
2. Fidget frequently	Research has shown that fidgeting, such as tapping toes and fussing with hands, blasts off up to 800 extra calories per day.
3. Get on top	Skip the passive missionary position and climb on top. This position decimates 4.5 calories per minute.
4. Take the stairs	Every minute you climb kills seven calories.
5. Take two	Taking the stairs two at a time burns 55 percent more calories than single stepping.
6. Rock out	Studies show that exercisers who tune in to music while exercising work out 25 percent longer.

Activity	Effort Expended
7. Give your lover a massage	An hour-long massage burns 230 calories.
8. Have sex	An hour of passionate playtime kills 270 calories.
9. Pace periodically	You could burn about 100 extra calories during an eight-hour day if you walk around your office, pace while on your cell phone or otherwise move around.
10. Kiss	Every minute you kiss someone you burn 1 calorie.
11. Don't order out	Cook at home. Spending an hour cooking burns about 150 calories. You can burn half of what you eat for dinner merely by cooking it yourself!
12. Sleep	You burn up to 200 calories while sleeping for around 7 hours.
13. Kick up your heels	Dancing burns 200 or more calories an hour, depending on the dance.
14. Do the hula hoop	This isn't just for kids anymore. In just 10 minutes you can burn 44 calories. Plus, you tone your tummy while doing it.
15. Jump rope	Fifteen minutes of jumping rope burns 170 calories.
16. Play with your kids	A game of hopscotch can burn 222 calories over the course of 30 minutes.
17. Coach your kids' sports team	Coaching burns between 281 and 372 calories an hour.

Review

- The Arrive Cycle is the weight-stabilization part of the 17 Day Diet.

- It provides a realistic way for you to manage your food and lifestyle.

- The foundational principle underlying the Arrive Cycle is to enjoy meal plans from one of your favorite Cycles—Accelerate, Activate or Achieve—from Monday through Friday lunch. Then Friday dinner through Sunday dinner enjoy your favorite foods and meals in moderation.

- Enjoy no more than one to three favorite meals over the weekend. Do not binge. Eat slowly and enjoy your food.

Angela James

"I'm much more comfortable in my clothes now."

AGE: **51**

POUNDS LOST: **12**

CURRENT CYCLE: **Arrive**

Angela, a PR agent in Los Gatos, California, had already finished cooking dinner for friends one night when she heard they had just started the 17 Day Diet. She had prepared barbecued meat with skewered vegetables and salad—and to her delight, this meal fit the plan perfectly! "Without knowing what I was doing, I had created a dinner that followed the diet. My friend was thrilled that she could eat everything I'd prepared." It wasn't long before Angela and her husband were trying the diet, too. After all, Angela says, "It seemed easy enough to be disciplined for 17 days."

At 5 feet 7 inches and 154 pounds, Angela was looking to drop a dress size and feel good about her body again. "I had hit a point where my midsection just wouldn't stop getting wider," she says. But once they started the Accelerate Cycle, Angela and her husband were each able to drop 12 pounds. "Within 17 days, I lost what I wanted to lose, and then I stabilized."

Angela's favorite part about her results is that she's back to her high school clothing sizes. "I was in a tight size 9/10, and now I'm in a comfortable size 7/8. This program slimmed me down and gave me energy back." The energy has been important in helping her keep up with her already active lifestyle—she's a member of two women's soccer leagues, she does Zumba twice a week, and she tries to take advantage of nearby hiking trails whenever she can. Even with all that movement in

(continued)

Angela James *(continued)*

her daily life, when the pounds continued to pile on, it was the diet that finally helped her reclaim her slender waistline.

"I learned that for me, the combination of foods allowed in the first 17 days was a great kick start and lasted just the right amount of time before I was able to introduce more foods. Although I am not watching my everyday diet as strictly now, I learned what I needed to succeed long term—and it has been an easy transition for me."

Angela progressed through Cycle 2 as directed, and then she relaxed a little more on Cycle 3. Now, on the final maintenance Cycle, she still relies on habits she picked up in the beginning: "I still do a probiotic serving twice a day, because I feel like that curbs my appetite for snacking," she says. She also sticks to fat-free dairy. "I got so used to it that I don't really see a difference. I'll use fat-free feta in salads and fat-free cream cheese in sauces. I incorporate it into our everyday life."

More than anything else, the plan has permanently changed her shopping habits at the grocery store. In addition to buying more probiotic yogurt products, she has made a lot of replacements, such as using lettuce to wrap burgers instead of buying hamburger buns. That trick also works for taco shells—she wraps the taco fillers and toppings inside large, sweet butter lettuce leaves. For Angela, making substitutions like these for flour-based foods is often one of the most challenging parts of staying true to the diet. However, finding a solution feeds her creativity, and she says it's rewarding to come up with substitutions that don't force her to cheat. Best of all, she has discovered a trove of new recipes. "One night, we were craving pizza. So I tried a cauliflower pizza recipe on one of the

17 Day Diet forums, and it was fantastic. I would never have tried that if I wasn't on the diet."

Angela turns to the forums on 17daydiet.com for all kinds of reasons, but most of all, she goes for the recipes. For example, she was able to find a 17 Day Dieter online who posted a modified version of *Dr. Mike's Power Cookie* recipe (page 266) to make a soft, rather than crunchy, cookie. Especially during the first 2 Cycles, this resource was a boon to Angela. "When I really couldn't figure out what to cook, I could go to the forum for a recipe or a fix." One of her favorite snack ideas is a vegetable dip with fat-free sour cream. "I always keep that dip ready so I can sit in front of the TV and crunch away."

Not only does she get to eat great food throughout the program, but Angela can rest assured that she's setting good examples about meal planning and food selection for her loved ones. "I went to visit my daughter at college last May, and she was bragging to her friends about the weight I had lost. My daughter has always been thin and fit, but she asked me to copy the meal planning pages out of the book and send them to her. She now tries to do a couple meals a day on the program."

Her advice:

- "When you do your shopping, stock your refrigerator all at once. Buy all the ingredients you'll need so that they are in easy reach when it's time to get cooking."

- "Also visit the forums. Reading about other people's experiences and how they cope with the recipes is very helpful."

PART II

. . . .

Special Considerations

7

The 17 Day
Cultural Diet

I look Italian. People think I am Italian, except of course for Italians, who think I'm from Brazil, Spain or Argentina. But my ancestry is Mexican; I was born and raised in the United States. Because of my origins, I'm able to relate to patients from many different cultures, and of course, because I speak Spanish, I can communicate with my Hispanic patients without an interpreter in the room.

Language issues are important in medicine. A lot of people who seek medical help can't speak English—and sometimes find themselves getting the wrong treatment, which can turn out to be both costly and embarrassing. We had a man once who was about to be treated for back problems. But he didn't have back problems, he had constipation. He was trying to refer to his "backside," but the nurse thought he meant "back." Or maybe he was too embarrassed to point to that part of his body.

In the nutrition area, I feel strongly that many people, due to their heritage, are not getting adequate nutritional counseling to lose weight. This is a big problem. When people come to the United States from other countries, they leave their traditional foods behind and adopt the Americanized diet that is high in carbohydrates, sugar and fat—often with life-threatening consequences. Among many Hispanics, for example, there exists a tendency to develop type 2 diabetes in their thirties and forties, about 10 years earlier than the average population, and it is triggered by weight gain, lack of exercise and smoking. Heart disease is another risk. But many of the dietary recommendations Hispanics in general receive in the United States do not conform to their beliefs about food or their cultural practices. The same is true for many other cultures.

I can't solve that problem in one chapter, but I'm going to give you a list of foods from your culture that you can eat on all four Cycles of the 17 Day Diet, if your heritage is Hispanic, Mediterranean, Asian, Indian or Persian.

Hispanic Cuisine

As I know from growing up, fried food, grease and salt are common ingredients in the typical Hispanic diet—and the cause of health-threatening disease in men, women and also children.

The good news is that if you are Hispanic, you don't have to turn your back on your ethnic favorites. You just need to challenge the food ingredients and preparation. Let's look at the food lists.

Cycle 1: Accelerate

Stick to the lists of approved foods, but add in these cultural selections:

Lean Proteins

Ceviche (white fish marinated in lemon juice with diced tomatoes, onions, chile peppers and cilantro)

Red snapper (huachinango)

Cleansing Vegetables

Concentrate on traditional favorites such as tomatoes, onion, summer squash, cauliflower, garlic, green beans and chiles (literally hundreds of varieties), tomatillos and cilantro

Cycle 2: Activate

Stick to the list of approved foods, but add in these cultural selections:

Lean Proteins

Reduced-fat chorizo

Goat meat

Natural Starches

All varieties of beans and legumes

Brown rice instead of white

Calabaza

Yucca (cassava root or manioc)

Arracache

Yautia

Plantains

Cycle 3: Achieve

Stick to the list of approved foods, but add in these cultural selections:

Lean Protein

Introduce Hispanic-style cheese known as queso fresco or "fresh cheese" as a protein. It contains less calories, fat and cholesterol than other cheeses such as cheddar, mozzarella or processed cheese products. It's not fake cheese either, thank goodness. My idea of hell is a place where Mexican food is made with artificial cheese.

Natural Starches
Low-carb tortillas

Corn (maize) tortillas

Bolillos (sour dough bread)

Cleansing Vegetables
Chayote

Jicama

Nopales

General Tips

- Many Mexican dishes such as beans, tortillas, Spanish rice and potatoes are good sources of carbohydrates. Beans are also high in fiber. But it is necessary to part company with tradition when it comes to frying or refrying. The time-honored method is to fry them in lard. Try boiling instead.

- Try preparing refried beans with less oil (use olive oil, not lard), or put them through a food processor and sauté them in a pan that has been coated with vegetable cooking spray.

- Scale back your intake of sour cream (try Greek yogurt instead). Or use salsa or pico de gallo to top your entrées.

- Reduce fat by using a variety of cooking sprays—and for much more than just sautéing. Try butter-flavored sprays for softening or baking tortillas, or olive oil sprays on grilled vegetables, fish or poultry.

- Use herbs and chiles in place of fats and oils.

- Use low-fat or fat-free cream cheeses. Fat-free cream cheese or low-fat ricotta lends a creamy texture to beans and sauces. Combine fat-free cream cheese and low-fat buttermilk to make a sour cream sauce. Avoid non-fat sour cream, which tends to have an offensive taste.

- Use low-fat cheeses in small amounts. They are tastier when mixed with highly flavored ingredients like chiles, spices and salsas.

- Instead of cooking tortillas in oil or other fat, brown them on the griddle and then oven-bake them a few minutes to heat the ingredients inside.

- Focus on eating simply prepared dishes flavored with traditional seasonings minus high-carb, high-fat sauces. Salsa is another favorite made from finely diced tomatoes, onions and chile peppers. This green or red chile sauce adds spice to a meal but not many calories. Many Hispanics are not used to eating foods without grease or salt. But with the right spices, the tastes can almost be duplicated.

Mediterranean Cuisine

There's actually no one "Mediterranean" diet. At least 16 countries border the Mediterranean Sea. The region's cuisines include Italian, Greek and Spanish foods. Diets vary between these countries and also between regions within a country. But the common Mediterranean dietary pattern has these characteristics:

- High consumption of fruits and vegetables

- High consumption of bread and other cereals, potatoes, beans, nuts and seeds

- Emphasis on olive oil as an important monounsaturated fat source (monounsaturated fat doesn't raise blood-cholesterol levels the way saturated fat does)

- Low-to-moderate consumption of red meat, fish and poultry

- Low-to-moderate consumption of cheese and yogurt

- Moderate consumption of red wine

Sounds healthy. Does a Mediterranean-style diet follow the 17 Day Diet recommendations?

Close, but not exactly. In general, the diets of Mediterranean peoples contain a relatively high percentage of calories from fat. This is thought to contribute to the increasing obesity in these countries, which is becoming a concern.

For the most part, the Mediterranean diet is fresh and flavored with garlic, onions, tomatoes and fresh herbs and other vegetables. It is, therefore, enormously rich in antioxidants.

Most of the foods on the 17 Day Diet are found in Mediterranean cuisine. Here are few to add in.

Cycle 1: Accelerate

Stick to the lists of approved foods, but add in these cultural selections:

Cleansing Vegetables

Broccoli rabe

Fennel

Italian flat-leaf parsley

Sugar-free marinara sauce (½ cup = 1 serving)

Cycle 2: Activate

Adhere to the list of acceptable foods, but add in these cultural selections:

Natural Starches

Orzo

Polenta

Risotto

Tabouli (Crushed wheat kernels that have been parboiled and mixed with chopped tomatoes, parsley, mint, olive oil and lemon juice)

Cycle 3: Achieve

Stick to the list of acceptable foods, but add in these cultural selections:

Natural Starches

Flatbreads made from white whole grain, whole wheat and multigrain

Whole grain Italian bread

General Tips

- Serve hot grilled chicken on a bed of steamed broccoli rabe sprinkled with lemon juice and pepper.

- Cook liberally with canned tomatoes. Cooked tomatoes provide more beneficial antioxidants, such as cancer-fighting lycopene, than raw tomatoes.

- Stay away from fat-laden butter sauces, and stick with tomato-based veggie sauces. The calorie count will be lower.

- Try sliced fennel sautéed over a little olive oil until translucent. Add cannellini beans, and top with a piece of salmon. Sprinkle with chopped Italian flat-leaf parsley for a great Activate Cycle meal.

- Use whole grain pastas, spaghetti squash or shirataki noodles (low-carb pasta) in place of regular pasta.

- Reduce the oil when making hummus and baba ghannoush, or delete it altogether.

- Dip sliced cucumbers in hummus rather than bread.

- Use whole grain pita bread rather than white bread.

- For a nutritious, high-fiber, low-fat lunch, try whole wheat pita bread stuffed with Greek salad.

- Heart-healthy main dishes include shish kebabs, souvlaki (Greek fast food consisting of small pieces of meat and sometimes vegetables grilled on a skewer), or plaki (fish baked or broiled with garlic and tomato sauce). Dolmas (stuffed vegetables) make an excellent choice because they are usually steamed or baked.

- For condiments: Certain spices that are popular in the Mediterranean diet—oregano, parsley and basil—can spice up your cooking, as can allium-containing vegetables such as onions and garlic.

Asian Cuisine

Asian diets are associated with the best life expectancy in the world. The longevity can be chalked up to a typical healthy, low-fat diet, which is widely believed to result in a lower frequency of heart attacks and strokes than in other countries. Asians also eat their meals at regular times, chew their food well, take in lots of fiber through vegetables and fruits and drink tea frequently. Here's how to adapt the 17 Day Diet to Asian dietary standards.

Cycle 1: Accelerate

Stick to the lists of approved foods, but add in these cultural selections:

Cleansing Vegetables

Arame, a form of kelp best known for its use in Japanese cuisine

Bamboo shoots

Bean sprouts

Bok choy

Chinese broccoli

Dulce, sea lettuce (used in many international cuisines)

Lily pods

Long beans (an Asian vegetable similar to domestic green beans)

Nori, an edible seaweed commonly used as a wrap for sushi

Pea pods

Snow peas

Cycle 2: Activate

Stick to the list of approved foods, but add in these cultural selections:

Lean Protein
Tofu, all varieties

Organic bison meat

Natural Starches
Brown rice rather than white rice

Edamame

Cycle 3: Achieve

Natural Starches
Add in the following starches (½ cup = 1 serving):

- Soba noodles: These distinctive Japanese noodles are made from buckwheat flour, but some wheat flour is usually added to strengthen the dough.

- Ramen noodles: Although associated with Japan, this style of curly wheat noodles (sometimes made with egg) actually originated in China.

- Rice noodles: As the name suggests, these delicate noodles, which are used throughout Southeast Asia, are made with rice flour.

- Chinese wheat noodles: A variety of noodles made from wheat and sometimes eggs.

- Udon noodles: A type of wheat-flour noodle popular in Japanese cuisine.

General Tips

- Boil, grill, steam or lightly stir-fry seafood, chicken, vegetable and tofu dishes—healthy techniques that require minimal fat.

- Try traditional steaming (often done over herb-scented water) in a multilayered bamboo basket. You can whip up several different fat-free dishes in one pot (less hassle and cleanup) in about 10 to 15 minutes. As a bonus, veggies, fish and other foods retain their shape, texture, flavors and nutrition.

- Don't deep fry. Use a non-stick pan and spray with vegetable spray as needed. You'll end up getting the same effect with a fraction of the oil.

- Avoid making thick sauces laced with "artery-popping" amounts of fat and sodium.

- Substitute tofu in recipes that call for eggs.

- Substitute turkey for beef whenever possible. Turkey has a lot less saturated fat compared to red meat. Eat more fish than meat.

- Enjoy green tea, recommended on the 17 Day Diet. It contains potent antioxidants that can lower cholesterol levels, fight heart disease, boost immune function and perhaps even destroy cancer and fat cells.

- For condiments, experiment with exotic fat-free flavors: lite soy sauce, fish sauce, oyster sauce, black bean sauce, miso (fermented Japanese bean paste that is a probiotic), seaweed, chiles, wasabi (Japanese horseradish paste), kimchi (a Korean condiment made from pickled cabbage that is a probiotic), curries (favored in Thailand), garlic, scallions, ginger, lemon grass, basil and cilantro.

- What about fortune cookies? Strictly an American invention.

Indian Cuisine

Generally, Indian meals are healthy and well-balanced. They're based on a variety of antioxidant-rich vegetables; meat, fish and poultry, when included, typically come in lean cuts and small portions. Vegetarian dishes are often the centerpiece of meals, too. Generally, the unique spices used in Indian dishes add flavor without fat. Here's how to adapt the 17 Day Diet to Indian dietary standards.

Cycle 1: Accelerate

Cleansing Vegetables
Sea vegetables such as arame, dulce and nori

Cycle 2: Activate

Natural Starches
Basmati rice

Red lentils

Cycle 3: Achieve

Natural Starches
Chapatis (unleavened flatbread made from whole wheat meal)

Any type of flatbreads made from white whole grain, whole wheat and multigrain

General Tips

- Vegetable curries, salads with raita (shredded vegetables) and lentils make great high-fiber additions to your meals.
- Try tandoori chicken or fish for a low-fat meal with a flavorful twist.
- Use yogurt in marinades as a tenderizer, along with ginger root, garlic and curry spices, for vegetables before grilling.
- Use yogurt, too, as a low-fat substitute for cream and a thickener for curries.
- Replace ghee, a clarified butter, with olive oil or flaxseed oil. There is also a cholesterol-free ghee.

- Spices are an integral part of Indian cooking and alleviate the need to cook with a lot of fat. Some of the most common digestion-enhancing spices include ginger, cumin, coriander, fennel, black pepper and cinnamon. Turmeric is ubiquitous in Indian cooking and is valued for its ability to stimulate digestion, improve liver function, enhance detoxification and bolster immunity.

Persian Cuisine

Although Persian cooking may seem exotic to Westerners, its presence is felt today in our own kitchens. When we cook with oranges, pistachios, spinach or saffron, for example, we use foods that originated in the region around Persia, now called Iran. When we use basil, cilantro, cumin and caraway, we are drawing on an age-old tradition of meatless cooking adopted by Persians from the empires of Sumeria, Babylon, Mesopotamia and Assyria.

Persian cuisine has undergone thousands of years of refinement but has never lost touch with its roots. The home of many common herbs, Persia was also the source of sweet and sour sauces, stuffed grape leaves, pastries and noodles. Some historians believe that pasta originated in Persia, not in Italy. Worth emphasizing too is that yogurt is used widely in Persian cooking.

Here's how to adapt the 17 Day Diet to Persian dietary standards.

Cycle 1: Accelerate

Stick to the list of approved foods, but add in these cultural selections:

Cleansing vegetables
Asian eggplant

Courgette (zucchini)

Grape leaves

Fruits

Persian lemon

Sour grapes

Cycle 2: Activate

Stick to the list of approved foods, but add in these cultural selections:

Fruits

Barberries, used in Persian cooking for their sour flavor

Pomegranate

Cleansing Vegetables

Yellow peas

Probiotics

Labne, a thickened yogurt made by straining yogurt in cheese cloth or a coffee filter overnight

Cycle 3: Achieve

Stick to the list of approved foods, but add in these cultural selections:

Natural Starches

Thin flatbread (lavash)

Non flatbread

General Tips

- Focus on traditional dishes like torshie hazeri (blends of vinegar or lime juice and vegetables), which lend themselves well to the 17 Day Diet. Another is sabzi khordan, a plate of raw greens—scallions and watercress, mint and basil—which are eaten with the fingers, or tucked inside lavash with a slice of feta cheese.

- Sauté vegetable mixtures such as borani with a minimum of oil, or use vegetable cooking spray and a non-stick pan.

- Make frittatas (kuku) with egg substitutes rather than eggs to cut calories and fat.

- Use brown rice instead of white rice in entrees.

- For probiotics, enjoy classic tzatziki, a yogurt cucumber dip made with yogurt, grated cucumbers and garlic.

Now You're Cooking . . . and Losing Weight

The 17 Day Diet works for everyone, no matter what your culture or country of origin. The main reason is that it encompasses mostly natural foods, and these are found in all cuisines. I think you have to use some food commonsense too: eating too many greasy tacos, deep-fried egg rolls or fat-laden pasta sauces can lead to more pounds, increased levels of cholesterol, clogged arteries and, ultimately, heart disease.

Fortunately, taking care of your body, health and heart doesn't have to mean giving up all your old traditional favorites. Just use low-fat cooking techniques, concentrate on fruits and vegetables in their most natural state and rely on probiotics like yogurt (which seems to be a staple in many cultures). Be innovative, use some ingenuity and apply some creativity, and you will lose weight.

Review

- The 17 Day Diet is adaptable to any cuisine. One reason is that it emphasizes vegetables, fruits, lean protein and whole grains—food groups that are a part of all cultures.

- Food preparation is key. Using less cooking fat and fewer starchy foods, you can make over many ethnic dishes to suit your diet.

- Be sensible: eat smaller portions and avoid frying or otherwise cooking foods in too much fat.

- The 17 Day Diet is for everyone, no matter what your cultural heritage or country of origin.

8

The PMS
Exception Diet

．．．．．．．．．．．．．．．．．．．．．．．．．．．．．

There's always an exception to every rule, but most of the time I
want you to follow them anyway. But premenstrual syndrome
(PMS) calls for bending the rules a bit.

Women, I'm sure you're happy and well-adjusted . . . until a few
days before your period, when you turn into Attila the Hun and snap
at everyone for no apparent reason. Your family and friends avoid you,
and who would blame them?

Next comes the physical stuff, like your body being so bloated that
it should be listed on MapQuest. Then, as your period arrives, so do the
cramps. For the next week, the love-hate relationship you have with
your period (you love that it comes regularly; you hate everything else
about it) turns hostile.

On top of all this, it's hard to stay on your diet. When you're not
doubled over with cramps, you're sticking your finger in a bottle of
hot fudge sauce multiple times a day or eating more in one meal than
Paris Hilton weighs.

We doctors still aren't positive why you might get testy as your
period rolls in, but the prevailing theory is that fluctuating levels of

estrogen and progesterone affect the mood-enhancing brain chemical serotonin. Serotonin is a chemical in your brain that, in proper levels, makes you feel happy. It's like a natural upper. When levels dip—which is what happens in PMS—you feel moody and crappy.

But here's the thing: you don't have to be a slave to your menstrual cycle. You can stick to a reasonable diet that one miserable week every month—and still lose weight. This is important, because being overweight or even obese makes PMS symptoms worse. You can accomplish this by following what I call the PMS Exception Diet. It's a combination of anti-PMS foods and supplements.

There are many lucky women who don't suffer from PMS and won't need this diet. The first step, before you consider this diet, is to determine: Do you suffer from PMS?

You might think that's a dumb question, and maybe it is. Most women know if they have PMS. Please humor me. We doctors went to school for eight years, and we like to put our medical training to use. We love asking questions to arrive at a diagnosis. Sometimes we even throw in unrelated questions, like "What kind of shampoo do you use?" or "Who played Carrie's California boyfriend on *Sex and the City*?"

Please take the following test. It will take just a second.

CHECKUP: Do You Suffer from PMS?

Do you have any of these symptoms right before and/or during your period? Check off any of the symptoms that apply.

☐ Depression	☐ Anxiety
☐ Headache	☐ Nightmares
☐ Food cravings	☐ Nausea
☐ Bloat	☐ Mood swings
☐ Cramps	☐ Breast tenderness
☐ Feelings of sadness	☐ Crying jags

☐ Desire to withdraw from social situations ☐ Irritability ☐ Fatigue	☐ Sleep disturbances ☐ Hot flashes ☐ Weight gain
It's easier to diagnose a broken arm than premenstrual syndrome, but if you have five or more of these symptoms, then you're probably suffering from PMS. Less than five, and you've probably got simple menstrual discomfort.	

Whether you have emotional symptoms or yours are more physical—cravings, bloating and back pain—PMS can seem like a necessary evil. But you don't have to put up with it. Armed with some cutting-edge nutritional info about this condition and a little planning, you can easily turn things around so that your period no longer has the upper hand in your life—and you can still lose weight, without blowing your diet. I'll show you how to take charge right here. First, we'll look at foods that help ease symptoms; second, foods that aggravate symptoms and should be avoided; and third, how to modify the 17 Day Diet for one week to help you continue losing weight.

MISTER MD, CAN YOU PLEASE TELL ME ❓

Aren't there any drugs my doctor can prescribe for my PMS symptoms?

Women have been suffering from PMS for years, and they are often treated with tranquilizers, antidepressants and diuretics. Over-the-counter painkillers like ibuprofen are effective against cramps. But honestly, simple changes in lifestyle (a healthy diet, exercise) have been found to be as effective as medication in eliminating symptoms.

Eat to Beat PMS

I give my female patients lists of recommendations, and I help them decide what to incorporate. Of all the changes you can make to improve your premenstrual health, physicians and nutritional experts agree that adopting healthful eating habits will have the most immediate effect. Here is an overview of what to include on the PMS Exception Diet.

Salmon and Other Fish

High in protein, fish like salmon, tuna, halibut, sardines, mackerel and herring are also high in beneficial omega-3 fatty acids, which can decrease cramps and other symptoms. These fats also stabilize the hormone spike that makes PMS so pronounced.

One of the fatty acids in the omega-3s is DHA, shorthand for docosahexaenoic acid. Low levels of DHA have been linked to depression. A study published in the medical journal *Lancet* stated that in regions where people ate more fish, there were fewer cases of depression. Another study, published in the *American Journal of Clinical Nutrition,* noted that the documented increase in depression in North America over the last century has paralleled the dwindling amount of DHA in our diets. Considering the evidence, I think it's a good idea to eat more fish. It seems to be a good natural treatment for depression.

Other gifts from seafood include calcium, magnesium, iron and zinc—all vital for easing symptoms.

One-Week PMS Exception Diet Prescription: Aim for at least 2 to 3 servings of seafood when experiencing symptoms.

Other Lean Proteins

Enjoying lean proteins such as lean meat and chicken helps you get selenium, an important anti-PMS mineral. Anxiety is associated with a deficiency in this mineral. Five weeks after psychologists at University College in Wales started administering a daily supplement of 100 micrograms of the mineral selenium to a group of 50 women and men, the subjects reported feeling more balanced and generally in higher spirits. Those most deficient in selenium at the start reported the most dramatic mood boost. The U.S. Department of Agriculture has reported similar findings.

Other sources of selenium are seafood (particularly tuna) and whole grains. You can meet your entire daily selenium requirement by eating three Brazil nuts a day.

Include the following proteins this week:

Chicken breasts

Lean beef

Lean ground beef

3 Brazil nuts daily

One-Week PMS Exception Diet Prescription: Enjoy at least 2 servings of lean protein daily. Have 3 Brazil nuts every day during your period.

Soy Proteins

Tofu, tempeh, soy milk and edamame (boiled, lightly salted soybeans in the pod) contain plant hormones called isoflavones, which may lessen PMS symptoms. There's evidence these natural compounds help your body absorb the extra estrogen and progesterone that play a role in making you feel moody, bloated and crampy.

One-Week PMS Exception Diet Prescription: Enjoy soy foods as snacks a few times a week during your period.

Natural Carbohydrates

Carbohydrates are the dietary building blocks of serotonin, that wonderful feel-good chemical in your brain. But not all carbs seem to be equally good at building serotonin. Many women with PMS report fewer symptoms after eating complex carbohydrates (whole grains, vegetables, fruit) because they are broken down more slowly by the body, keeping blood sugar, and possibly the source of serotonin, steady. Simple carbohydrates (sugar, syrup, honey) boost your blood sugar and serotonin levels only temporarily, so after an initial high or calm, you may feel irritable or moody. Alcohol (think of it as super sugar) may have similar effects.

Carbs such as lima beans and black beans are high in potassium and magnesium—two minerals that help prevent mood swings, fatigue, cravings and bloating. Sweet potatoes are rich in B vitamins, a family of nutrients that help curb PMS symptoms too.

One-Week PMS Exception Diet Prescription: Include 3 daily servings of the following:

½ cup cooked oatmeal

1 cup high-fiber cereal

1 slice whole grain bread (no sugar added)

½ cup beans or legumes

1 medium sweet potato

½ cup corn

½ cup barley

½ cup brown rice

Water-Flushing Vegetables

A number of foods are thought to be diuretics, meaning they help the body eliminate water. And most contain magnesium, potassium, calcium and other nutrients that can relieve PMS. Asparagus, by the way, is one of the best. It contains an amino acid called asparagine that (bonus!) acts as a diuretic to flush excess liquid out of your system. Vegetables are also full of fiber, which aids elimination and relieves abdominal bloating.

Eat the following vegetables during your period:

Asparagus

Beets

Cucumbers

Lettuce, all varieties

Parsley

Spinach

Tomatoes

Watercress

One-Week PMS Exception Diet Prescription: Eat water-flushing vegetables liberally each day.

Higher-Sugar Fruits

Like certain vegetables, many fruits are loaded with potassium, an anti-PMS nutrient. Some honorable mentions: banana, cantaloupe, grapes and mangoes. Yes, these fruits are high in sugar, but that's a plus on this plan. Fruit is nature's candy and will help tame sugar cravings during your period.

Steer toward high-fiber fruits too, such as apples, pears and berries. Eat your fruit instead of drinking it, since fruit juice is almost pure sugar.

One-Week PMS Exception Diet Prescription: Enjoy up to 3 servings of fresh fruit daily, with an emphasis on the fruits discussed above.

Probiotics and Calcium-Rich Foods

You're already eating probiotics on the 17 Day Diet. Well, guess what? These good bacteria can keep you regular and bloat-free. In one study, women with abdominal pain, bloating, constipation and/or diarrhea who took the probiotics in supplement form for four weeks noticed less bloating than those on a placebo.

Probiotic foods, such as yogurt, supply an important anti-PMS mineral: calcium. Research shows that women who consume 1,000 to

1,200 milligrams of calcium a day all month have fewer menstruation-related mood swings than do those who skimp on dairy products. A calcium deficiency seems to make hormone fluctuations worse, so getting enough of this mineral keeps hormones steady and serotonin high. You'll feel significantly less nervous, irritable, depressed and moody.

One-Week PMS Exception Diet Prescription: Enjoy 2 servings of probiotics daily. Choose from the 17 Day Diet lists.

Anti-PMS Fats

Your body needs essential fatty acids (EFAs) to efficiently metabolize hormones. EFAs are a collection of polyunsaturated fats vital for bodily functions. "Essential" means that our body is unable to manufacture it, and we need to draw it daily from our diet.

To be of benefit to your body, EFAs are converted to prostaglandins. Prostaglandins are hormone-like substances responsible for the regulation of blood pressure, dilation of blood vessels for better circulation, prevention of clotting of the blood, reduction of inflammation and regulation of insulin levels. They also act as a watchdog of the immune system.

Supplementation with EFAs that contain a fatty acid called gamma-linolenic acid (GLA) and/or omega-3 fats has been shown to be useful in the management of PMS symptoms. Evening primrose oil is high in GLA and is an effective anti-PMS supplement that can be taken in capsule form (see page 191). Flaxseed oil is loaded with omega-3s and is thus a great fat to eat during your period. It assists in hormonal regulation.

One-Week PMS Exception Diet Prescription: Have 1 to 2 tablespoons of flaxseed oil daily as your friendly fat serving. Talk to your doctor about taking supplemental fats.

Chocolate

The recommendation to eat a bit of chocolate during your period is controversial. Some docs say okay; others say no. I'm among those who believe that chocolate is the antidote for grumpiness. Everyone gets happy when they eat chocolate. It actually boosts the brain's production of serotonin, and chocolate contains phenylethylamine, the same brain chemical that occurs in higher concentrations when you're in love.

Chocolate has many other virtues. It's rich in magnesium, a calming mineral. If your relationship with chocolate is based on health benefits, the darker the better. Dark chocolate has the highest cocoa content, and cocoa is the magic stuff; it's rich in flavonoids, a group of chemicals that protect the heart and blood vessels from tissue damage. (Milk chocolate is typically sweeter and less intense than dark chocolate, but much lower in flavonoids.)

So go ahead, let chocolate make your day, but limit daily consumption to about ½ to 1 ounce of dark chocolate or some low-calorie cocoa. Of course, use moderation if you feel the urge—no eating both ears off a 6-foot chocolate bunny. Any benefit of chocolate will be wiped out if you gorge on it and gain weight. Don't deny your cravings during your period, but control them.

One-Week PMS Exception Diet Prescription: Enjoy ½ to 1 ounce of dark chocolate or some low-calorie cocoa during the week of your period, if you have a craving for chocolate.

Other Nutritional Tips to Fight PMS

Multiple meals. Aim to get five to six meals daily (breakfast, lunch, dinner and snacks). The point is to maintain a steady blood-sugar level. A steady intake of foods high in complex carbs helps keep blood sugar high, so you're less affected by the hormone-induced irritability. Try not to go more than three hours without eating. Meals with a good balance of natural carbohydrates and a moderate amount of protein seem to do the trick for many women.

Water your body. To avoid bloating, some women steer clear of extra water right before their periods. Putting more fluid into an already bloated body seems like the last thing you'd want to do, but in fact, drinking water is one of the best ways to stimulate your body to get rid of excess fluids. (If you avoid water, your body responds by hoarding fluids, making bloating even worse.) So drink at least eight cups of pure water a day.

What to Avoid

A number of foods and substances will make your symptoms worse. Avoid the following.

Soda. You don't drink this on the 17 Day Diet, and you definitely don't want to drink it during your period. The bubbles in carbonated drinks will make your belly pooch out. Stick to plain water.

Gum. Chewing gum causes you to swallow excess air, and this aggravates bloating. So when someone says you're full of hot air, you are. Spit your gum out.

P.M. Carbs. On the 17 Day Diet you don't eat carbs past 2:00 p.m. anyway. This is a good practice to follow during your period. Starchy foods like bread and pasta may cause you to retain water. Lay off them before bedtime to keep from waking up puffy.

Salt. Even a few shakes can be enough to promote bloating and breast tenderness. Cutting back on salt is a pretty easy change to make, and it can really help with your symptoms. Spice up foods with herbs, spices, low-sodium or no-salt seasonings, low-salt soy sauce, sea salt or kelp.

Caffeine. Foods and beverages containing caffeine can increase breast tenderness, anxiety, irritability and mood swings. Caffeine can also rob the body of B vitamins, which are important for keeping hormone levels in balance. Recent studies found that the more coffee a woman drinks, the worse her PMS conditions are. Don't cut back on caffeine too drastically, or you may suffer withdrawal symptoms. Trim your coffee intake by a half cup every few days, or mix regular with decaffeinated, gradually upping the proportion of decaf over several weeks. Also begin easing up on other sources of caffeine, such as some teas and colas.

Refined sugar. It's a no-no. White sugar hampers the absorption of magnesium, an important nutrient; causes large fluctuations in blood-sugar levels, which can make you feel fatigued; and robs

MISTER MD, CAN YOU PLEASE TELL ME ❓

My digestion is so out of whack during my period. What can I do?

What you're describing is fairly typical. Poor digestion can actually worsen PMS, so take the following precautions:

1. Eat a variety of whole foods to ensure you get all the nutrients you need. Avoid canned, frozen and otherwise processed foods.

2. Eat freshly prepared foods whenever possible.

3. Eat your heaviest meal around noon. The later in the day you eat, the lighter your meals should be. This helps with weight control too.

4. Chewing your food thoroughly makes it easier to digest.

5. When preparing meals, create a peaceful, relaxed atmosphere in your kitchen to infuse your food with a healthful energy.

6. If possible, eat at the same time every day.

7. Eating warm or hot food promotes better digestion.

8. Don't drink cold beverages; they decrease the digestive power in your stomach. Try drinking plain hot water flavored with freshly squeezed lemon juice.

your body of B vitamins. Stop stuffing yourself with sugar-laced comfort foods when you're feeling low. You'll feel much better if you steer clear of sweets. The immediate lift provided by sugar is usually followed by fatigue, and if you're already susceptible to depression, then being tired may make things look worse than ever.

Alcohol. Limit your intake to no more than one drink a day, or none at all, during your period. It can act as a depressant and make you irritable.

Eggs. During your period, pass up eggs in favor of egg whites. The fat content in eggs can interfere with the absorption of magnesium.

The PMS Exception Diet

Here's a look at an effective way to plan your meals during your period. Use these sample meals as a guideline to plan your own week of symptom-free living.

Day 1

Breakfast

- Cinnamon apple oatmeal: Peel and dice or grate 1 medium apple. Cook the apple with oatmeal (to yield ½ cup of oatmeal). Serve and sprinkle with cinnamon. Cinnamon helps stabilize blood sugar.

Lunch

- Turkey sandwich: On 2 slices whole grain bread, spread a tablespoon of Dijon mustard and top with slices of low-fat turkey breast and tomato slices.
- 6 oz. fat-free plain or sugar-free yogurt with 1 cup diced mango

Dinner

- Grilled salmon

- Large salad of lettuce, tomatoes and parsley, drizzled with 1 tablespoon flaxseed oil and 2 tablespoons herbed vinegar

Snacks

- 3 Brazil nuts

- 1 oz. dark chocolate

- 6 oz. fat-free plain or sugar-free yogurt, or 1 cup soy milk

- ½ medium cantaloupe

Day 2

Breakfast

- Cheesy parfait: Combine ½ cup Breakstone's LiveActive cottage cheese with 1 cup berries (any variety) and 3 chopped Brazil nuts

Lunch

- 1½ cups whole wheat pasta (this constitutes your 3 servings of natural carbs for the day) topped with sugar-free marinara sauce

- 1 medium apple or pear

Dinner

- Grilled or baked chicken

- Plenty of steamed asparagus

- Sliced tomato, drizzled with 1 tablespoon flaxseed oil and herbs

- ½ cup low-fat chocolate pudding

Snacks

- 6 oz. fat-free plain or sugar-free yogurt

- 1 medium banana

Day 3

Breakfast

- 1 cup cocoa made with soy milk
- 2 scrambled egg whites
- 1 slice whole grain toast
- ½ medium cantaloupe

Lunch

- Tuna sandwich: Mix a 3 oz. can of tuna with 1 tablespoon light mayonnaise and 3 tablespoons finely diced celery. On 2 slices whole grain bread, spread tuna mixture and top with tomato slices.
- 6 oz. fat-free plain or sugar-free yogurt with 1 cup diced mango

Dinner

- Grilled steak
- Large salad of lettuce, tomatoes and parsley drizzled with 1 tablespoon flaxseed oil and 2 tablespoons herbed vinegar

Snacks

- 1 medium apple or pear
- 3 Brazil nuts
- Large bowl of edamame

Day 4

Breakfast

- 1 cup high-fiber cereal
- 1 medium banana, sliced and placed on cereal
- 1 cup soy milk

Lunch

- Large spinach salad with spinach leaves, topped with ½ cup tofu (cubed), 2 slices cooked turkey bacon, crumbled, ½ cup garbanzo beans and chopped parsley, drizzled with fat-free dressing
- 1 slice whole grain bread
- 6 oz. fat-free plain or sugar-free yogurt with 1 cup fresh berries

Dinner

- Grilled pork chops
- Cucumber and tomato salad: Slice half a cucumber, combine with a cup of grape tomatoes, and drizzle with 1 tablespoon flaxseed oil and 2 tablespoons herbed vinegar.

Snacks

- 3 Brazil nuts
- 1 oz. dark chocolate
- 6 oz. fat-free plain or sugar-free yogurt
- 1 medium apple or pear

Day 5

Breakfast

- Cheddar melt: Top 2 slices whole grain bread with 3 tablespoons shredded reduced-fat cheddar cheese. Broil in toaster oven until cheese melts.
- 1 cup melon balls

Lunch

- Chef salad: Large bed of lettuce, chopped cucumber, ½ cup garbanzo beans, sliced pickled beets and strips of baked chicken or turkey drizzled with 1 tablespoon flaxseed oil and 2 table-spoons herbed vinegar

- 6 oz. fat-free plain or sugar-free yogurt with 1 cup fresh berries

Dinner

- Grilled or baked salmon
- Steamed asparagus
- ½ cup low-fat chocolate pudding

Snacks

- 1 cup fresh pineapple chunks
- 3 Brazil nuts
- Large bowl of edamame

Day 6

Breakfast

- Smoothie: In a blender, combine ½ cup soy milk, 6 oz. light or fat-free plain yogurt, 1 banana, sliced, a dash of vanilla extract and 4 ice cubes.
- 1 slice whole grain toast

Lunch

- Boiled or steamed shrimp
- ½ cup lima beans
- ½ cup corn
- 1 medium apple or pear

Dinner

- Grilled steak
- Mixed green salad with parsley, chopped cucumbers and grape

tomatoes, drizzled with 1 tablespoon flaxseed oil and 2 table-spoons seasoned or balsamic vinegar

- 1 5 oz. glass red wine

Snacks

- 3 Brazil nuts
- 1 oz. dark chocolate
- 6 oz. fat-free plain or sugar-free yogurt
- ½ medium cantaloupe or 1 cup strawberries

Day 7

Breakfast

- 2 scrambled egg whites
- ½ cup oatmeal
- 1 cup berries

Lunch

- Lean hamburger patty
- 1 cup brown rice
- Stewed tomatoes
- 6 oz. fat-free plain or sugar-free yogurt
- 1 medium apple or pear

Dinner

- Roasted turkey breast
- Steamed asparagus
- Cucumber and tomato salad: Slice half a cucumber, combine with a cup of grape tomatoes and drizzle with

1 tablespoon flaxseed oil and 2 tablespoons seasoned
vinegar

- 1 5 oz. glass red wine

Snacks
- 3 Brazil nuts

- 1 oz. dark chocolate

- 6 oz. fat-free plain or sugar-free yogurt

- 1 medium banana

Supplement Savvy for PMS

The pills I do like to throw at medical problems are nutritional supplements. There are many supplements you can take on a regular basis
that can help. Consult your doctor about considering the following:

Multivitamin/mineral. Take one in the morning with food. (If taking
children's vitamins, take 2 tablets.) Taking a multi with food
optimizes the absorption of the vitamins and minerals, especially B6, magnesium and potassium—nutrients that help ease
premenstrual distress. Vitamin B6 is important for helping the
liver regulate excess estrogen levels and has been shown to help
prevent menstrual cramps.

Vitamin D. Sufficient daily intake of vitamin D (400 IU) might also
alleviate PMS symptoms, particularly irritability.

Calcium carbonate. At least 1,200 milligrams. The average woman's
diet provides only 600 to 800 milligrams of calcium a day, not
the 1,000 to 1,200 mg necessary to ease PMS symptoms. One
study found that women who took this dose had a 48 percent
drop in the severity of their PMS symptoms. Calcium appears to
enhance the brain's processing of serotonin.

Magnesium. 400 milligrams twice daily. This mineral has a calming effect and counteracts irritability. Whole grains and lentils are loaded with it, but you can also get it in a supplement. Magnesium may improve mood, and one study has shown it can provide significant relief to women suffering from menstrual headaches. Magnesium citrate, aspartate and glycinate are better absorbed than the oxide form.

Fish oil. 3 grams daily. Up your dosage to 5 grams daily when PMS symptoms begin.

Evening primrose oil. 1,000 milligrams daily. It relieves one of the most common PMS symptoms: breast tenderness.

If the changes I'm recommending seem too daunting, try making just a few at a time. My patients tell me that eating more regularly, eliminating refined sugar and caffeine, plus exercising more, make the biggest difference. Or target your most bothersome symptoms: If your breasts really bother you, for example, try taking evening primrose oil or cutting out salt to see if you get relief.

To assess whether the PMS Exception Diet is working for you, you really have to try it for at least 6 cycles. Keep notes. As your symptoms decrease, you'll be motivated to stick to your new plan. If a symptom persists, or you keep gaining weight, consult your doctor. Keep in mind your ultimate objectives: relief of PMS symptoms and ongoing weight loss.

Review

- Several minor adjustments in the 17 Day Diet can help you during your period. Include more omega-3-rich foods such as salmon, increase your daily intake of natural carbs to 3 servings a day, eat more water-flushing vegetables and enjoy higher-sugar fruits.

(continued on page 194)

LEAN 17: 17 Bloat Busters

t's Saturday night, and you slip on your sexiest pair of jeans. One problem: Your stomach is so swollen that those jeans barely zip. Sound familiar? Bloating is a common but annoying PMS symptom with many causes. Fluid retention in women is frequently due to the hormonal changes that happen right before your period arrives. There are brain hormones and brain chemicals that affect the gut; estrogen and progesterone are actually brain chemicals. They affect the brain and nervous system, and have an effect on the motility, or movement, of the gut. Luckily, there are easy ways to banish bloat, about 17 in all. Try one of these tricks to keep your denim from fitting a little too close for comfort.

1. Stop eating high-sodium stuff like canned soups, fast food and cured meats. Sodium causes your body to hang on to water.

2. Drink more water. Believe it or not, extra fluids will help to flush out the sodium—and the bloat.

3. Avoid simple carbs (think white bread, white pasta, chips, etc.). Carbs get broken down into glucose and stored in the body as glycogen for energy. In order for the glucose to be stored, a water molecule must attach to it. The more stored carbs you have, the heavier you'll feel.

4. Opt for high-fiber carbs like vegetables and fruit. The longer food sits in your intestines, the more likely you are to retain water.

5. Exercise. It sweats out excess water and speeds up digestion. When you exercise, you stimulate the muscles that help move food and water through your system faster. Fight constipation by walking for at least 17 minutes each day to keep food moving through your digestive tract. Working up a sweat also releases fluids. In addition, research shows that moderate exercise soothes cramps, headaches and lower-back pain, improves sleep and reduces fatigue. And exercise boosts endorphin levels, which helps improve your mood.

6. Take calcium and magnesium, as I mentioned above. Both compete with sodium for absorption into your body, so if you take in adequate amounts of either, your body is forced to flush out the salt that wasn't effectively absorbed.

7. Be wary of diuretics. When you stop taking a diuretic, your body retains more water, making you bloat for one to two weeks afterward. This can lead to a physical dependency so that your body needs the drug to rid itself of the excess fluid instead of doing it naturally.

8. Shun sodas. I just cannot overstate this recommendation. The caffeine in sodas dehydrates you, and phosphorus, a common soda additive, can inflame your intestinal wall, making you feel even puffier.

9. Discuss the appropriateness of birth control pills with your physician. Birth control pills may stabilize your level of progesterone, a bloat-inducing hormone.

10. Boost your B_6. Many PMS symptoms, including water retention, are triggered by a defect in your body's metabolism of vitamin B_6. Take 50 to 100 milligrams of B_6 daily to see if it helps.

11. Stop the junk. Reduce your intake of foods that are difficult to digest, such as sugary, fatty and fried fare, which can sit in your gut, causing constipation and distention.

12. Enjoy water-flushing vegetables.

13. To beat bloat, try a natural diuretic drink, such as a cup of chamomile or dandelion tea or a glass of noncarbonated water with lemon or lime.

14. The artificial sweetener sorbitol, found in some sugarless gums and candies, can contribute to bloating, as can the consumption of alcohol, caffeine and even nicotine.

15. Also avoid dairy products that contain lactose—milk sugar—if they seem to worsen your bloating symptoms.

16. Up your protein the week before and during your period. Protein has a diuretic effect on the body.

17. Take supplemental probiotics.

- Probiotics and calcium-rich foods help with digestion problems and mood swings.

- Eat a bit of chocolate during your period. It helps with stress relief.

- Eat multiple meals (5 to 6 daily) to maintain a steady blood-sugar level.

- Avoid soda, chewing gum, p.m. carbs, too much salt or caffeine, refined sugar and eggs.

- Several supplements can help: a multivitamin/mineral, vitamin D, calcium, magnesium, fish oil and evening primrose oil.

- Employ bloat-busting strategies, including drinking lots of water throughout the day.

THE 17 MINUTE WORKOUT: Sunlight Soothes PMS Symptoms

Outdoor aerobic activity is best if you're trying to alleviate PMS discomfort. Sunlight has been shown to reverse depression, carbohydrate cravings, fatigue and irritability in women with PMS. Spending too much time indoors under artificial light can make PMS symptoms worse.

So try some brisk walking, playing tennis, running, hiking or biking. These are all activities that contribute to a heightened sense of relaxation and well-being. Aerobic exercise, in general, elevates the production of endorphins—brain chemicals that have a soothing effect. It also helps keep your heart and bones healthy and relieves muscle tension.

In addition to regular aerobic activity, the next best exercise prescription for PMS includes yoga to stretch muscles, align the spine and increase mental focus. But don't overdo exercise, since excessive exercise causes irregular periods or the cessation of menstruation and unhealthful conditions that can lead to the premature loss of bone.

PART III

. . . .

Make It Stick

9

Dining Out
on the 17 Day Diet

No one stays home anymore. Where are we? We're sitting in restaurants. On average, Americans dine out four times a week, according to the National Restaurant Association. As we eat out more and more, the percentage of obese people increases, while their wallets decrease. We spend $1 billion a day dining out. The Census Bureau's population clock has the U.S. at 310,751,194 people, so if we spend some $365 billion a year eating out, that averages out to $1,117 per person per year, a large portion of which could be savings if you ate at home instead.

Yikes! I guess you have to ask yourself if you want to be overweight or rich.

When we dine out, most of our meals don't even include a cloth napkin because we're eating at fast-food joints. Fast-food restaurants are everywhere, even in hospitals. That means you can get your high-fat, high-calorie fast food and your medical care in the same place. Unfortunately, your insurance company does not reimburse you for these meals.

Hospitals claim these restaurants are not for patients, but for the visitors and employees. Sure. Anyone who works in a hospital knows that a lot of that food will be smuggled into patient rooms. When you're sick in bed in the hospital, you know who your true friends are and they're not bringing flowers and balloons.

Hospitals have gotten savvy in other ways. Did you know some even offer "room service"? That's right. Meals are served bedside by waiters in a black tie and crisp burgundy jackets. This makes you feel like you're in a restaurant, only you're lying on your back in a hospital gown, staring up at the ceiling and developing a new appreciation for acoustic tile.

"Hi, my name is Walter and I'll be your waiter."

Just when you think you get to place an order for filet mignon, garlic mashed potatoes and cheesecake, Walter says:

"Would you like red, green or yellow Jell-O with your meatloaf?"

Your heart sinks and you reluctantly say, "Red Jell-O."

Regardless of where you eat out (hospitals or otherwise), you might be surprised to see just how high the calorie counts on some restaurant meals are. A healthy-sounding chicken fajita omelet at IHOP, for instance, weighs in at 1,360 calories. (According to the Food and Drug Administration, recommended daily calorie intakes for adults run from 1,600 to 2,800 calories a day.) So eating that omelet takes a huge bite out of your recommended calorie intake.

What if you opt for the more "healthful" carrot cake over the cheesecake at the Cheesecake Factory? Oops. As per the company's materials in early 2011, one carrot cake slice offers 1,549 calories. Consider a Taco Bell Chicken Ranch Taco Salad with salsa in a shell: 910 calories and 55 grams of fat. Ouch. Or a medium-size Starbucks mocha coffee accompanied by a cinnamon chip scone has a whopping 770 calories, 30 grams of fat.

These numbers aren't exactly trade secrets. You can find them on the restaurants' websites, but in the next few years, they will start showing up on their menus as well, thanks to a small provision in the massive health care law signed in 2010. The new rule applies to restaurant chains with 20 or more locations.

On the next page is a look at more calorie surprises.

Unrestrained, this type of eating out is the perfect recipe for obesity and disease down the road. But we've trained ourselves to eat out. We're just too busy to cook.

So what's the answer? Eat only steamed veggies? Refuse to dine out? On the contrary. You can dine out successfully on the 17 Day Diet

LEAN 17: The 17 Most Fattening Restaurant Choices

Menu Item	Calories*
1. Cheese fries (4 cups with 8 tbsp. ranch dressing)	3,010
2. Bloomin' Onion	2,400
3. Fried seafood combo platter (with 4 tbsp. tartar sauce, fries, coleslaw and 2 biscuits with 2 pats of butter)	2,170
4. Fried chicken dinner, with a biscuit and mashed potatoes	2,000
5. Combo lo mein noodle dish	1,820
6. Kung Pao chicken with rice	1,600
7. General Tso's chicken with rice	1,600
8. Fettuccine Alfredo	1,500
9. Cheesecake	1,500
10. Molten chocolate cake with ice cream	1,270
11. Spaghetti with meatballs	1,200
12. Beef and broccoli with rice	1,200
13. Stuffed potato skins (8 skins with 5 tbsp. sour cream)	1,120
14. Lo mein	1,100
15. Fast-food shake, large	1,010
16. Fried calamari	1,000
17. Cheese quesadilla or chicken burrito	1,000

*Calorie counts at particular restaurants may vary.

and enjoy your experience by learning how to navigate any menu. These days, more restaurants than ever offer low-fat, low-cal menu items, making it easy to enjoy a delicious, nutritious dining experience, if you know what to ask for. Let me offer some tips that will help you eat smart while dining out.

Know Before You Go

With most restaurants these days, you can go online and look at their menus. See what dishes look healthy—grilled items, salads, vegetable sides, and so forth. Decide before you go what you'll order, and stick to your decision once you get there. Collect the menus in the restaurants you frequent so that you have them to refer to.

Sit in a Quiet Spot

Nobody knows this, but people who sit in the more distracting parts of restaurants (by a window or in front of a TV) eat considerably more. Commotion makes it easy to lose track of how much you're putting in your mouth. If you're making a reservation, request a quiet table. If you walk in and are offered a table in a busier spot, ask for one away from the action. It's worth the wait.

Be the First to Order

You've decided to pick something light off the menu, but when your friend orders the decadent steak frites, you start to rethink your boring grilled salmon. To sidestep the temptation of your friend's less healthy dish, place your order first. If you can't order first, then make your decision, close the menu, and repeat your selection to yourself to help you stick to it. If you're dining at a restaurant you visit often, just ask for your favorite healthy option without ever opening the menu.

Have It Your Way

Before ordering your selections, ask the server about the details of the meal. This will help you make more informed choices. Some questions to ask include:

- How is this dish prepared? Can it be modified?
- What ingredients are used?
- Do you have any low-fat or low-calorie options?
- What comes with this meal?
- Can I make substitutions?
- How large are the portions?

Don't be afraid to make special requests. For example, ask that foods be served with minimal butter, margarine or oil. Ask if a particular dish can be broiled or baked rather than fried. Also, ask that no additional salt be added to your food.

You may also be able to make substitutions. If the ingredients are on the menu, the chef should be able to accommodate your needs. A common substitution is a baked potato for fries, or a double serving of vegetables instead of a starch. If your dish does not arrive at the table the way you ordered it, don't be afraid to send it back.

If you don't see something you like, ask for it. As a paying customer, you have the right to eat not only what tastes good, but what's good for you. Be "weight assertive"!

Don't Be Seduced by Menu Descriptions

Mouth-watering descriptions like "tender, juicy chicken breast" or "ripe heirloom tomatoes" are increasingly common on restaurant menus. Be extra aware of sensory terms like "velvety" mousse and nostalgic ones like "legendary" spaghetti and meatballs. Research shows that words that promote taste and texture or appeal to diners' emotions can increase sales by 23 percent, and can even influence the way you think the food tastes. Words like these prep your taste buds to expect your chicken to taste juicy, so to some degree it probably will.

Make a game out of picking the colorful adjectives on the menu. See who can find the most in three minutes. If you win, everyone buys you dinner. That's the rule of the game.

Stay Away from Snacking

The most damage often occurs before the actual meal begins: appetizer trays are loaded with fat. Besides that, they take away your appetite for the healthiest foods to come. Avoid them. Even the freebies like chips and salsa at Mexican restaurants or a basket of rolls and butter at other establishments can pile up fat and calories that you don't need. If you can't exercise control, have your server remove the temptation.

Make a Meal out of Appetizers

Certain appetizers can be excellent choices for an entrée. The portion size of appetizers is often more appropriate than the extremely large portions provided in entrées. Consider healthful options such as steamed seafood (for example, shrimp cocktail), salads that aren't loaded with high-fat ingredients (such as cheese and bacon), grilled vegetables and broth-based soups. You might also choose to combine the appetizer with a salad; the salad will bulk up the meal so that you feel more satisfied without adding a lot of calories. Be aware that some appetizers, particularly fried fare or items covered in cheeses, oils and cream sauces, may be overloaded with calories and fat. Some fried appetizers can provide a day's worth of fat to four people!

Be Salad Savvy

A salad can be your meal's best friend or worst enemy, depending on how you toss it. Pile on fresh greens, beans and veggies, but don't drown it with high-fat dressings or toppings like cheese, eggs, bacon or croutons. Pick calorie-friendly dressings (vinaigrettes, low-cal dressings, even a generous squeeze of fresh lemon).

Remember, too, that you can gain control over the fat and calories in your salad by ordering the dressing on the side. Measure out a small amount of dressing with your spoon, or with thicker salad dressing, use the fork-dipping method. Dip the tines of your salad fork in the dressing, then spear the leaves of your salad. That way, you get a taste of the dressing with each bite of salad.

If you want to be really "good," carry one of those salad spritzer products in your purse. Order your salad without dressing. Pull out your spritzer and spray your salad. Be aware, though, that this might scare the other patrons, who will think you are sanitizing your salad.

And watch out for potato salads, macaroni salads, coleslaw and even tuna and chicken salads, which usually are heavy in mayonnaise, sugar and calories.

Go Low on Sides

Depending on which Cycle you're on, substitute high-cal side dishes with low-fat options such as steamed vegetables, brown rice or fresh fruit. Forget the French fries, and have baked, boiled or roasted potatoes, but leave off the butter, cheese and creams. Flavor with salsa or pepper and chives instead.

Choose Low-Fat Preparation Methods

The way your entrée is prepared influences its calorie and fat content. Choose grilled, broiled or baked meats and entrées. Pan-fried and deep-fried foods give you extra fat you don't need. Broiling, baking, steaming, poaching and grilling seafood, skinless poultry, lean meat and veggies give you all the flavor without all the fat.

For example, grilled chicken is lower in fat and calories than fried chicken. (If you are served chicken with skin, you can remove the skin to save significant fat and calories.)

It's not easy to get rid of all fat in restaurant meals, but give it a try. Ask the server if the butter or oil used to prepare your entrée can be reduced or eliminated. Even a grilled item may have extra fat added. For example, some grilled beef dishes call for added oil.

Enjoy Alcohol in Moderation

Drinks can be diet-killers, too. Ice water is free, but fancy mixed drinks have lots of empty calories, and the alcohol can dull your reasoning. Since alcohol can contribute significant amounts of calories, limiting your intake to 150 calories' worth is a good idea. The following portions of alcohol each contain 150 calories or less:

5 oz. of wine

1.5 oz. of liquor

12 oz. of light beer

Many people find it helpful to order wine by the glass rather than the bottle so that they can better control and monitor their intake. You can decide ahead of time at which point in the meal your beverage would be most satisfying. For example, you may want to save your glass of wine for your entrée and sip water while you wait for your meal. Holding off on alcohol until a later course also helps to decrease alcohol's effect on your inhibitions. If you drink alcohol on an empty stomach, it can relax you to the point that you lose sight of your game plan. Setting a personal limit and planning when to enjoy your beverage should help you stick with your goals.

Practice Portion Control

Restaurants serve mountains of food—about two to three times the quantity that we need in a meal. This is no big secret. Just don't try to finish those mega-size portions. Consider sharing a meal or taking a doggie bag so that you can have a quick meal at a later time. Eat until you're satisfied, not stuffed, and take the rest home. As you're eating, use my Hunger/Fullness Meter, listen to your internal hunger signals and stop when you have had enough. Eating slowly helps you recognize such cues.

Keep track of how much you eat, and stick to the number of servings you planned to eat. You probably won't bring a scale with you to the restaurant so that you can measure out portions, but you can rely on visual references. For example:

- A serving of cooked meat, chicken or fish is like the palm of your hand, or about the size of a deck of cards.
- A serving of green salad is like an open-cupped hand.
- A serving of fruit or vegetables is like your fist, or about the size of a tennis ball.
- A serving of baked potato looks like a baseball.
- An ounce of cheese is like your middle and index fingers together, or about the size of four stacked dice.
- A serving of salad dressing is like your thumb.
- A 3-ounce hamburger patty is the size of a quart-size mayonnaise jar lid.

Practice the Three-Bite Rule

Try to satisfy your sweet tooth with fresh fruit, and that's it. Wave off the dessert cart. Don't even order dessert, unless you're on Cycle 4 and are enjoying "weekends off."

That said, you can also practice my three-bite rule with desserts, if you want to watch your calories a little more strictly.

There are lots of variations on the three-bite rule, by the way. Moms try the three-bite rule all the time. "Johnny, you must eat at least three bites of everything on your plate before you're excused from the table." This usually does not work. Mothers spend many long, painful, tearful hours in a standoff, while kids discover at least 152 ways to say "disgusting."

My variation on the three-bite rule is different. If you truly want chocolate turtle cheesecake, go ahead and have it, but limit yourself to a taste. Take three bites and then set it aside for a few minutes. You're less likely to come back to it. You might even discover that those few bites of a great dessert can be very satisfying, and might be all you really wanted in the first place. You can't possibly blow your diet big-time on three bites of anything. After your three bites, you can ask your server to take it away, unless your dinner mates want to scarf it down.

Incidentally, servers use the three-bite rule all the time. After they serve the food, they wait until you have had three bites. Then they come back and ask if everything is okay.

If you're being good on your diet, you will ask the server to remove the rest of the dessert. Be careful here. This may hurt the server's feelings. You have to soften the blow by explaining that you, too, are practicing the three-bite rule.

Choose Wisely at Any Meal

Looking for more healthy ideas while dining out? These general suggestions can help you make good choices at almost any restaurant.

Breakfast

Cereal with skim milk topped with fruit

Oatmeal with fruit or raisins and skim milk

Wheat toast

Eggs, Egg Beaters or egg whites (including omelets)

Low-fat or "light" yogurt

Fresh fruit

Appetizers

Gazpacho or vegetable juice

Broth, bouillon or consommé

Vegetable soup without cream

Shrimp cocktail

Steamed clams or mussels

Green salad (without meat or cheese) with dressing on the side

Vegetables

Steamed, stewed, boiled or grilled vegetables without butter or sauces

Starches

Baked or boiled potatoes

Pasta or steamed rice (whole wheat pasta and brown rice are preferable)

Entrées

Lean meats: grilled, broiled or served au jus (trim excess fat)

Fish or skinless poultry: grilled, steamed, baked, broiled or poached in wine, lemon juice or lime juice (all without added fat)

Ahi tuna

Beverages

Water, mineral water, seltzer, tea or coffee (unsweetened)

Virgin Bloody Mary

Glass of dry red or white wine

Fast-Food Choices

Grilled chicken sandwiches, hold the bun

Entrée salads

Movie Snacks

Kid-sized box of popcorn

Bottle of water

Dill pickle (Yes, many movie theaters serve these. But be careful
   when you bite down or else you will spray pickle juice on the
   head of the guy in front of you and create a commotion.)

Here are some other ways to choose wisely at just about any restaurant.

Best Choices at Ethnic Restaurants	
Asian	• Steamed rice
	• Steamed Chinese vegetables
	• Stir-fry vegetables with shrimp/chicken
	• Teriyaki beef or chicken
	• Steamed or baked tofu (make sure it is not fried) and vegetables
	• Hot-and-sour soup
	• Miso soup
	• Entrées made with chicken or fish and vegetables
	• Steamed chicken and vegetables with a half cup of brown rice

	• Any boiled, steamed or lightly stir-fried seafood, chicken, vegetable or bean curd dishes • Sushi • Sashimi • Edamame
Delicatessen	• Half a deli sandwich—roast turkey with mustard on rye • Lox with tomato and onion • Low-fat deli meats, such as low-fat turkey or even low-fat ham • Salad with dressing on the side • Whole wheat bread, rye or pumpernickel
French	• Poached fish entrées • Roasted or grilled lean meats • Bouillabaisse • Nicoise Salad • Broth-based soups • Plain vegetables
Greek/Middle Eastern	• Yogurt-based dips • Meat and vegetables on a skewer • Grilled meat entrées • Stuffed pepper with meat and rice • Cabbage rolls • Tabouli • Vegetable dishes and soups

(continued)

Indian	• Any dish with beans, rice, grains or vegetables
	• Chicken tandoori
	• Vegetable curry
	• Shrimp bhuna
	• Fish vindaloo
	• Lentil soup
	• Salad or vegetables with yogurt dressing
Italian	• Minestrone
	• Vegetable antipasto
	• Mussels with marinara sauce
	• Chicken marsala
	• Clams with marinara sauce
	• Spaghetti squash with marinara (some Italian restaurants have this variety of squash on their menus; it makes a delicious, low-calorie substitute for pasta)
	• Chicken cacciatore
	• Veal piccata
	• Grilled chicken or fish entrées
Mexican	• Grilled foods such as chicken or fish
	• Salsa
	• Pico de gallo
	• Tortilla soup
	• Black or red beans
	• Black bean soup
	• Mexican rice
	• Chili with beans
	• Salad, dressing on the side

Stay healthy but leave room to be flexible when you eat out: eating is an integral—and fun—part of life, and life can be unpredictable. An unexpected change in your daily eating plan isn't the end of the world. In fact, you can enjoy dining out even more if you remember that it's your total diet that counts, not individual meals. You're always going to eat out at restaurants. Hopefully, you'll eat a little differently most of the time.

Review

- Be prepared before you go out to eat at a restaurant. Check out online menus and decide what you will order.

- Sit in a quiet spot (people eat more in noisy restaurants) and be the first to order, so that you're not influenced by what your friends order.

- Be assertive with the wait staff. Ask how foods are prepared, and request that your order be made according to low-fat, low-calorie preparation methods.

- Make a meal out of appetizers, since appetizer portions are often smaller than entrées.

- Order salad dressing on the side, or bring your own.

- Enjoy alcohol in moderation, since it can increase your appetite and lower your inhibitions.

- Practice portion control. Don't eat the whole thing; take some home for lunch or dinner the next day.

- Try the three-bite rule, especially for desserts.

CHECKUP: DR. MIKE'S RESTAURANT QUIZ—How Much Do You Know about Nutrition at Popular Restaurants?

f you're trying to reduce the calories and fat in your diet, dining out can be a challenge. Take my quiz to test your restaurant smarts.

1. Which 6-inch sandwich at Subway has the *fewest* calories?

   A. Subway Club

   B. Tuna Salad

   C. Roast Beef

   D. Steak and Cheese

2. Which breakfast item at McDonald's has the *most* calories?

   A. Steak, Egg, and Cheese Bagel

   B. Hot Cakes with syrup

   C. Egg McMuffin

   D. Sausage Burrito

3. Which salad at Subway has the *most* calories?

   A. Black Forest Ham Salad with Fat-Free Italian Dressing

   B. Turkey Breast Salad with Fat-Free Italian Dressing

   C. Sweet Onion Chicken Teriyaki Salad with Fat-Free Italian Dressing

   D. Veggie Delite Salad with Fat-Free Italian Dressing

4. Which of the following from TCBY has the *fewest* calories?

   A. ½ cup of no-sugar-added vanilla frozen yogurt

   B. ½ cup of orange sorbet

5. Of the types of pizza you can order at Pizza Hut, which variety has the *most* calories (based on ⅛ medium 12-inch pizza)?

   A. Cheese Pan Pizza

   B. Medium Cheese Thin N Crispy Pizza

   C. Hand Tossed Cheese Pizza

   D. Veggie Lover's Pan Pizza

6. What is the average calorie count of a 20-ounce Stay Healthy smoothie at Smoothie King?

   A. 362 calories

   B. 248 calories

   C. 422 calories

   D. 195 calories

7. Which muffin at Dunkin Donuts has the *most* calories?

   A. Corn Muffin

   B. Coffee Cake Muffin

   C. Blueberry Muffin

   D. Honey Bran Raisin Muffin

8. What is the *lowest*-calorie plate you can order at Boston Market?

   A. Baked Whitefish

   B. Beef Brisket

   C. Half Rotisserie Chicken

   D. Pastry Top Turkey Pot Pie

9. What is the average calorie count of a seafood entrée at Captain D's Seafood?

   A. 223

   B. 758

   C. 589

   D. 350

10. Which 16-ounce drink at Starbucks has the *most* calories?

    A. Hot Chocolate

    B. Flavored Latte

    C. Cappuccino

    D. Caffe Mocha

(continued)

How did you do? The answers may surprise you:

1. The correct answer is C (Roast Beef) at 310 calories. The Subway Club sandwich weighs in at 320 calories; the Steak and Cheese sandwich, 380 calories; and the Tuna Salad sandwich, 530 calories.

2. The correct answer is A (Steak, Egg and Cheese Bagel). It has 660 calories. Hot Cakes have 530 calories. The Egg McMuffin and the Sausage Burrito have 300 calories each.

3. The correct answer is C (Sweet Onion Chicken Teriyaki Salad with Fat-Free Italian Dressing) at 235 calories. The Black Forest Ham Salad and the Turkey Breast Salad with Fat-Free Italian have 145 calories each. The Veggie Delite Salad contains 85 calories.

4. The correct answer is A (½ cup no-sugar-added vanilla frozen yogurt) at 80 calories. The ½ cup of orange sorbet contains 100 calories.

5. The correct answer is A (a slice of Cheese Pan Pizza) at 240 calories. The slice of Medium Cheese Thin N Crispy Pizza has 190 Calories; the slice of Hand Tossed Cheese Pizza, 220; and the Veggie Lover's Pan Pizza, 230 calories.

6. The correct answer is C (422 calories). The lowest-calorie smoothie in the Get Healthy category is Blueberry Heaven at 325 calories; the highest-calorie smoothie is the Kiwi Island Treat at 498 calories.

7. The correct answer is B (Coffee Cake Muffin) at 630 calories. The Corn Muffin has 490 calories. The Blueberry Muffin and the Honey Bran Raisin Muffin have 480 calories each.

8. The correct answer is B (Beef Brisket, 4 ounces). It has 230 calories. The Baked Whitefish has 470 calories; the Half Rotisserie Chicken, 640 calories; and the Pastry Top Turkey Pot Pie, 790 calories.

9. The correct answer is A (223 calories). Seafood entrées range from 28 calories for 4 Scampi Shrimp to 770 calories for ½ pound of clams at this restaurant.

10. The correct answer is A (Hot Chocolate) at 300 calories. The Flavored Latte has 250 calories; Cappuccino, 120 calories; and Caffe Mocha, 260 calories.

Source: Nutritional guides at restaurants, as of early 2011.

THE 17 MINUTE WORKOUT: Burning Off a Super Burger

Super burgers at fast-food joints can rack up almost 600 calories a serving. Here's a look at how you can burn all that off.

- Participate in a 90-minute aerobics dance class (five 17-minute cycles).
- Jog for four 17-minute cycles.
- Ride a stationary bike vigorously for four 17-minute cycles.
- Shovel snow or dig ditches for three 17-minute cycles.
- Walk moderately for eight 17-minute cycles (about 2½ hours).

Wouldn't it be easier NOT to eat the super burger?

Source: Calculations are based on research data from *Medicine and Science in Sports and Exercise,* the official journal of the American College of Sports Medicine.

10

Family Challenges

Being on the 17 Day Diet can be satisfying and morale-boosting, especially as the pounds melt off. But do you ever wonder how your diet might affect the people seated across the dinner table from you? You know, your loveable hubby picking at his baked chicken breast and green beans, missing the old days when lasagna wasn't banished from the kitchen?

A study published a few years ago in the *Journal of Nutrition Education and Behavior* shed some light on the plight of the dieter's significant other. Researchers interviewed 21 pairs—mostly spouses and one father-daughter duo—to understand how one person's decision to lose weight or eat healthier food affected a partner.

The good news is that for the most part, significant others saw themselves as positive influences on a partner's battle of the bulge. Other partners, however, acted more like saboteurs, refusing to alter their junk food habits, and in some cases, offering little more than snide comments. A few were openly skeptical and critical of a partner's ability to succeed.

Bottom line: your loved ones—your husband, wife, kids, even your mother—may try to entice you to go off your diet even after you've made it very clear you're on it. And they may not even realize they're doing this.

There are a couple of reasons why this happens. A big one is jealousy. One person may fear that the relationship could change as a partner's waistband gets smaller, confidence grows and social life changes. It could scare your spouse that you're losing weight and developing a

Sabotaging Remarks and How to Respond

Don't be caught off guard by someone's remarks. Here are some suggestions for responding:

Saboteur: You're wasting away. Are you sure you aren't losing too much too fast?

You: It seems that something about me being slim is concerning you (or frightening to you or upsetting to you). But for me, my weight loss is a good and healthy thing.

Saboteur: Are you sure you can eat that?

You: My diet is varied and healthy. I eat foods in smaller portions. (Or, if such comments persist:) Until we can communicate about my food plan in a way that feels good to me, I don't want to discuss my diet anymore.

Saboteur: You don't like my brownies all of a sudden?

You: I like your brownies very much. But I'm not hungry right now; I'm full. (Or ask to wrap up some brownies to take home, but then toss them out.)

Saboteur: Here, one doughnut left, want it?

You: I really am working hard. I'm feeling great, and it would be nice to have your support. Is there anything I can do to help you give me that?

Saboteur: It's your birthday. One piece of cake won't hurt!

You: Yes, I know. I'm just so full . . . I'm going to take it home for later.

Saboteur: It's great you're losing weight. I hope you can keep it off this time.

You: You may feel that your comments about my weight are supportive, but it would help me if . . . (fill in the blank with something like "you didn't remind me of my past diets").

Saboteur: It's none of my business, but don't runners get a lot of knee injuries?

You: You know, I've spoken to my trainer, and my exercise habits are healthy.

Saboteur: Are you still on your diet? Have you lost any weight?

You: I appreciate your questions, but I might take them as pressure and feel frustrated if I can't report better numbers every time you ask me.

Saboteur: You know, you don't seem to be the same since you lost weight.

You: I really feel confused by that comment; I really want you to be supportive of my accomplishment.

kick-ass body. He might fear that other men will find you attractive, and you'll leave.

Another is fear of change. People don't want to change the status quo in their relationship. Couples often have unspoken contracts that they never articulate. For example, "If you don't bug me about my weight, I won't bug you about your drinking. If you don't bug me about my weight, I won't bug you about smoking. If you don't bug me about my weight, I won't bug you about sex." Then the wife decides to lose weight, and suddenly the husband says, "Oh, my God, I'm going to have to stop smoking."

People who sabotage do things like the following: Your partner might sit down and eat a bag of cookies right in front of you. Or refuse to touch your low-fat cuisine and demand that you fix cheeseburgers. Or offer glasses of wine and cheese and crackers, and you fall off your weight-loss wagon night after night. Or assign himself as the watchdog of your eating habits, telling you what to eat. This controlling attitude might backfire, making you rebel and eat more (especially if he's not eating the same healthful way). It's nearly enough to end your commitment to diet and exercise, especially when someone's actions feel like personal attacks.

Of course, it's not just spouses or significant others who can throw a wrench into healthful eating regimes. Office mates or friends can be just as destructive. Often, colleagues or friends who have been unsuccessful in their own efforts to lose weight, or office mates who are competing professionally, will be unsupportive. Even so, the biggest challenges come from right under your own roof—from your family—so that's who I really want to focus on here. Finding ways to get a partner on board is important because such support can play a major role in whether you succeed or fail.

Being the only one dieting in your family is a tough situation to be in. You make up your mind—no potato chips or chocolate ice cream in the house. No more temptations, because you're determined to change your habits and lose weight. But from talking to patients who want to lose weight, I say that's often only half the battle.

For those trying to drop pounds or eat healthier, the other half—the more trying half—can be resisting your loved ones' attempts to thwart your newfound resolve. Here are some thoughts I have on the subject.

Limit Exposure to Guy Food

Are you newly married? Some newlyweds are surprised to find out that not only do their new husbands own Bart Simpson bubble bath, but also they love junk food, and lots of it. Ice cream. Potato chips. Foods that you may have forgot existed, because as a single gal, you often subsisted on the four basic food groups: Weight Watchers, Lean Cuisine, Healthy Choice and Slim-Fast.

Exposure to guy junk food can tear down your defenses, even if you're just trying to lose 10 pounds on the 17 Day Diet. And from experience being a guy, I can tell you, many men do eat differently than women. The stereotypical guy eats heavy, fattening food. But it is possible to lose weight while living with a man.

I believe you must set firm ground rules, like the fact that certain foods are out of bounds, period. Give your husband a special shelf (preferably one you can't reach) to stash his junk food. Or ask him to hide it. Out-of-sight, out-of-mind is one of the best ways of coping. Okay, every now and then, you might find some Oreos in strange places, like under the sofa pillows.

Eat Less Than He Does

Men eat more than women. It's just a fact; we eat like linemen. Even the Feds have studied this: According to government surveys, the average American man 20 to 59 years old eats 2,758 calories a day, while the average American woman 20 to 59 eats 1,834 calories a day—about a third less. If you try to keep up with him, you'll keep putting on weight. Stop matching him bite for bite (you might not even know you're doing it). Always eat less than your husband does, particularly when dining out. At restaurants, immediately put one-half of your meal to one side and bring it home in a doggie bag.

Exercise While He Watches TV

Not only do we eat like linemen, we like to watch linemen on TV. Whenever you get the chance, put some exercise equipment in front of the TV and do a half hour on the stepping machine or stationary bike while he's watching sports. This strategy will help you get thin and stay that way.

Take Charge of the Kitchen

If your husband doesn't believe in, or think he likes, low-fat, low-cal eating, don't worry. You can fix healthy foods, and he'll never know the difference (except if his pants start getting mysteriously too baggy and loose). Instead of using all ground beef, use half ground turkey and half beef with spaghetti, for example. Make pasta with fresh vegetables. Cook vegetarian chili with tons of vegetables and beans; just don't call it vegetarian. Use cooking spray to sauté foods; it's a great way to cut down on the fat and calories. Done correctly, with the right food substitutions, low-fat meals taste as good as—and sometimes better than—their fattening counterparts.

Become Fitness Pals

In all seriousness, the best strategy is to get healthy and fit together. As any expert will tell you, it's much easier to eat healthy, nonfattening food if everyone around you is too. You can make a big deal out of each other's success, congratulating yourselves the whole time. Enjoy mealtime conversations again, instead of wolfing down food. Work out together. Invite your spouse or partner to try exercising, try this diet, or try healthy food. Phrase it lovingly: "I want to spend more time with you because I love being together. Let's do an exercise program together, like some couples training or couples yoga, or let's start bike riding after work. Wouldn't that be a great opportunity to be together more often?"

The decision to get fit together marks a good time to rethink your definition of love and affection. Sometimes spouses who do most of the cooking feel that they are expressing affection by piling rich food on your plate. To resist might be translated as rejection. You've got to renegotiate here. Explain that healthy cooking accomplishes the same end: Healthy cooking = love. Your "reformed" spouse will see that coming up with nonfattening meals is a bigger present than loading you up with junk, especially when he sees all the weight you're losing and how wonderful you look. Maybe someone should think of adding a line to the wedding vows: "For richer, for poorer . . . for skinnier and chubbier . . ."

By sharing the health and fitness experience with a partner, you can help each other stay motivated. Partners encourage one another to move from healthy to unhealthy behaviors. One study found that women who work out with their husbands are more likely to stick to fitness programs than married women who exercise alone. Another found that men are three times more likely to stay on a healthy diet if their wives encourage them to do so.

Sharing the fitness experience gives you something to talk about. Better communication, especially in loving relationships, is always a source of greater closeness.

Find Other Supporters

If you've tried your best but can't get your husband or partner on board, seek help elsewhere, such as with a friend, a coworker, other family member, or hire a personal trainer. They can give you encouragement and inspiration. If you don't get any takers, join a group, such as a walking club or a local yoga class. These activities are fun, and you get to meet more fitness-minded people that way.

Having positive support helps you reach your dieting and fitness goals. A team effort works more harmoniously. With two or more of you working together, there's more stamina, and more motivation to get to your goals.

No matter how challenging your situation, stay focused and remember your reasons for wanting to get slimmer and healthier. Imagine if someone told you that you could live longer and have less pain in your life. Would you listen to what they had to say? Exercise and healthy eating is as close to the fountain of youth as we have today.

Review

- Being on a diet affects the people around you. It's important for your success to bring them on board.

- Be prepared to respond to saboteurs.

- Negotiate the presence of junk food in the house with your spouse and other family members.

- Take charge of your kitchen and learn how to cook healthy meals that everyone in your family will love.

- Invite your spouse or partner to join you in your effort to get more fit.

- Build a support group of other fitness-minded people.

MISTER MD, CAN YOU PLEASE TELL ME **?**

I live alone and sometimes it's hard to stay on a diet. What suggestions do you have for me?

Single-person households have grown from 7 percent in the sixties to 27 percent of the total today. Many single diners are deficient in calcium, iron and other important vitamins and minerals because they skip meals, snack for dinner or open the freezer and prepare whatever falls out. Research shows that people who live alone are more likely to have vitamin and mineral deficiencies. Eating alone can be a pleasurable and healthy activity, if you plan your life around it. Some suggestions:

- Stock your kitchen with a variety of staples with a long shelf-life, such as brown rice, oatmeal and other whole grains.

- Keep on hand pre-chopped broccoli, bagged lettuce, and yogurt, so you don't use time as an excuse not to prepare foods.

- Make single dish meals with all the components—grains, meat and vegetables—such as in casseroles and soups. Prepare them ahead of time and freeze them so you don't have to cook a lot. Also, you can make the whole recipe but portion it into individual bags.

- Take advantage of supermarket salad bars. They're a boon to single people who may have avoided fresh fruits and vegetables they couldn't use fast enough. Skip the mayonnaise-based salads and high-fat dressings, but load up on fresh vegetables and fruits. At home you can add some low-fat meat or cheese, tuna or kidney beans and your own favorite low-fat dressing.

(continued)

- Never underestimate the uses of your freezer and microwave. Bags of frozen vegetables can be a great alternative when fresh produce is not available. Rice and pasta leftovers are particularly good candidates for freezing and later use. Use your microwave for defrosting and reheating, or to speed preparation of almost any meal. Microwave dishes often can be prepared with less fat, too, by adding bouillon, wine or broth.

- Dinner should be pleasant, and atmosphere does contribute to a more enjoyable meal. Set the table with linens, attractive dinnerware and a centerpiece. Make a lovely meal with fresh ingredients and enjoy it with a little wine, some jazz on the stereo and a couple of candles. Sit at the table; don't just eat hanging over the sink.

- If you're single, try to get together with friends on a regular schedule. Set up a Thursday night supper club and rotate homes or try a new restaurant once a month.

- Start a cooking club. Or have a standing date to eat potluck with friends once a week or month.

- Get together with a friend who likes to cook, and make a whole week's worth of good food that you split.

- Use the 17 Day Diet delivery service and get single serving meals delivered directly to your home.

- Don't be afraid to eat out alone. I eat out most meals and love experimenting. I'm quite oblivious to other diners so I don't mind being stared at. I simply open my iPad and scribble, which grabs the attention of the waiters, who think I'm a food critic.

11

Surviving Holidays

The holidays. It's the time of year when the zipper on your dress and the springs in your bathroom scale start getting really nervous.

That's because, for a lot of dieters, packing on pounds can be a holiday tradition. Statistics on weight gain throughout the holiday season assert that you might gain five pounds if you don't keep your hands off the pumpkin pie and figgy pudding.

I started thinking about this: A five-pound weight gain is a lot of food, if you consider that it takes 3,500 calories to gain a pound. This means you'd have to have major pig-outs on a daily basis or eat several reindeer at a buffet. You'd also have to spend the entire holiday season on the couch.

Still, it's easy to gain weight over the holidays, if you figure that the traditional holiday dinner with appetizers can weigh in at more than 3,000 calories!

How about this year we change that tradition? Commit to a holiday in which you manage not to gain any weight back before it's time to resolve to lose all that weight (and so much more) yet again.

Incidentally, by "holiday," I'm talking about everything that happens from Thanksgiving to Easter, including the sweetheart of all weight-gaining holidays, Valentine's Day. Holidays, however, do not include 99-cent Big Mac Mondays.

Okay, with all the office parties, cocktail receptions and dinner celebrations, can you eat, drink, be merry, stay fit and still follow the 17 Day Diet?

Answer: Absolutely—by adhering to my easy-to-follow holiday strategies. If you do, there will be no need to make a get-fit New Year's resolution, ever again. You'll start every year in super shape.

"Pre-Diet" Before the Holidays Hit

To prevent packing on holiday pounds, go on the offense with "pre-dieting." It works like this: Use the Accelerate or Activate Cycles to start trimming off a few pounds of fat before the holidays get in full swing. You can do this easily with what you've already learned from the 17 Day Diet.

Pre-dieting has been shown in clinical trials to offset holiday weight gain. Obesity researchers in Sweden studied the effect of eating during the Christmas holidays on 46 obese patients in a weight-maintenance program. Those dieters who had lost more than 6.6 pounds by pre-dieting during the six months prior to Christmas gained less weight (from 0.4 pounds to 4.8 pounds) between Christmas and Epiphany (a religious festival celebrated on January 6) than those who didn't pre-diet. By contrast, the patients who gained more than 6.6 pounds during the six months prior to Christmas put on an additional 5 pounds on average during the holidays. The message is clear: Pre-dieting clearly keeps the holiday pounds from piling on.

Don't resort to any type of crash dieting, however, in which you fast or slash calories down to 700 or less a day. This can result in a loss of muscle, decreased strength and power, low energy, moodiness or irritability and compromised immunity. Stick to the Accelerate or Activate Cycles for best results.

Party Plans

The hardest part, I think, is all those parties and dinners.

During the holidays, food is everywhere. Office parties, tins packed with homemade cookies, and holiday fruitcake offer little escape. Not only is there more food, but it's often rich in calories, sugar and fat.

Here's what I advise for enjoying yourself, without packing on any extra pounds.

- Continue the good habit of eating breakfast during the holidays to help control cravings later on. (Sorry, eggnog isn't considered a good egg substitute.)
- Have healthy snacks on hand. Go for them before you treat yourself to the splurge stuff.
- Eat a healthy dinner before you go to a holiday party. (Also, try not to eat an unhealthy dinner when you're at the party.)
- Prepare and take your own safe, low-calorie and low-fat foods to parties. That way you have at least one healthy alternative.
- Choose two or three of the healthiest appetizers you can find (a little shrimp, some veggies or fruit, etc.) and put them on a small plate or napkin, then walk away from the table. (Keep in mind this should be two or three pieces of food, not two or three napkins or plates loaded with food.)
- Be smart at the buffet table. Fill three-fourths of your plate with vegetables and fruits, the rest with protein. (Pumpkin pie and chocolate-covered strawberries don't count as the veggies or fruit. Stacking things as high as you can is not an acceptable method for filling your plate.) Do not circle the food table like a vulture. Serve yourself, and then go sit down somewhere to eat.

- Avoid temptation. Just say "no" to packaged holiday candies and cakes! Re-gift them to someone who's not dieting.

- Stay away from places where snacks and goodies are offered or stored—like the break room at work or the pantry at home.

- Give yourself permission to enjoy a little of everything that is usually only available during the holidays, but to do it in moderation. Indulging in small amounts of holiday treats (fruitcake being the exception) might not help you lose 20 pounds over the holidays, but it might help keep you from raiding the Christmas tree for edible ornaments in the middle of the night.

- Bank your calories. Accumulate a deposit of uneaten calories on the days when you know that you will be attending parties or enjoying holiday feasts. Eat a light breakfast and lunch to save calories for later. If you're careful, the large "withdrawal" of calories at a big dinner or event later on won't break the bank.

- Be extra good on non-party days.

- Understand the reason for the season. The holiday season is a time to celebrate good times with family and friends. Try to make the focus more on socializing, and less on eating.

Fill Up on Fiber

There's an incredibly easy, no-willpower way to stay lean during the holidays, something that most of us should be doing all year but aren't: eating more fiber. Increasing your fiber intake will help to transform your holiday dieting efforts into something simple and automatic. You'll be able to keep your weight under control without working at it or driving yourself crazy.

Fiber makes you feel full, so you're less likely to stuff yourself on high-calorie foods. What's more, the fibers found in foods such as bran, whole wheat products and oats naturally bind to the fats you eat and help to escort them from the body. The net effect is a reduction in the number of calories left behind that can be stored as body fat.

So fill up on legumes, fruits and vegetables.

Manage Alcohol Consumption

At holidays, alcohol flows like lava. Keep in mind that beer, wine and hard liquor are high in calories, however. In fact, each gram of alcohol has 7 calories, compared to 4 calories per gram for other carbs. Alcohol also stimulates your appetite. Remember too, when there's alcohol in your system, the liver has to work overtime to process it, so it doesn't have adequate time to process fat. A study conducted at the University of Lausanne in Switzerland found that the addition of only 3 oz. of alcohol per day to the diet resulted in about one-third less fat being processed.

You can avoid drinking alcohol and still remain social by sipping on seltzers, club soda or sparkling mineral water on the rocks with a citrus twist. Or opt for nonalcoholic beer or wine. But don't overdo it, because most of these products are high in sugar.

SCIENCE SAYS: Log What You Eat, Lop Off Pounds

During the holidays, keep track of what you eat and how many calories you consume daily by writing the information down in a food journal. Technically referred to as "self-monitoring," this practice has been shown in research to promote weight loss, even during the holidays.

In one study, 38 dieters (32 women and six men) recorded their food and calorie intake during Thanksgiving, Christmas or Hanukkah, and New Year's Eve. The researchers categorized the dieters into groups according to how consistently they kept track of their food and calorie consumption. Weight loss was recorded as well. The best and most consistent self-monitors lost an average of 10 pounds more than the persons who had a low level of compliance with the monitoring program.

Fit In Exercise

The holidays are not a time to take a vacation from your workouts. Stick to your regular exercise routine. It's one of the best ways to fight fat gain during the holidays. So regardless of what comes between you and your workout, try not to eliminate it altogether. If you're like most people, you'll need to let off some steam during the often-stressful holiday season, and exercise is the perfect stress reliever. Plus, it helps to burn off the extra calories that you've eaten at those parties and holiday get-togethers.

If you have the luxury of time during the holidays, why not engage in a little additional aerobics to burn off those extra calories? Do a bit more of your usual aerobic activity or try some new types just for fun. Spend an afternoon at an ice or roller-skating rink. Whack a ball around the racquetball court. If the weather permits, hit the ski slopes, try your hand at cross-country skiing or rent some snowshoes and go exploring.

If you're not that adventurous, try to slightly increase the duration and/or frequency of your usual aerobic exercise routine. Duration refers to the length of time that you work out. It's amazing how many additional calories you'll consume by pushing your body just a little longer.

Another option is increasing exercise frequency: working out more times per week to incinerate more calories and fat. Add some extra weekly sessions to your normal exercise routine.

Beef up your intensity. Make the effort count. For optimum fat-burning, you should exercise at a level that is hard enough to raise your heart rate to 70 to 80 percent of your maximum heart rate. (You can calculate your desired heart rate by subtracting your age from 220 and multiplying that number by 70 or 80 percent.) As an added bonus, exercising at a higher intensity has also been shown to suppress hunger.

So don't plop down on the sofa this holiday season—move your body!

Get a Grip on Holiday Stress

I've always thought the concept of "stress" attached to the word "holiday" was the ultimate contradiction. Shouldn't a holiday be simply filled with joy and celebration?

Yes! Even so, there is holiday stress, much of it self-imposed. What is supposed to be a time of joy and good cheer begins to resemble frantic preparations for a military invasion.

Along with the season's celebrations come temptations and preparations that can cause stress and fatigue. It's no wonder people often gain weight during this time of the year. To help you avoid the season's pitfalls, namely weight gain and stress, I'll give you my thoughts on how to organize your life to make time for what really matters. Don't let your holidays be downers. With some organization and planning, you can sail through the season with your health and emotional well-being intact, and maybe even a few pounds lighter.

- Manage your time and priorities. To prevent being hijacked by the demands of the season, do some planning. Decide which events and activities are most important and mark your calendar accordingly, along with planning for some "personal" time. Holidays are about family and friends, so decide which people are the most important (like family, close friends and those visiting from out of town), and spend more time with them. Gift buying and sending out holiday cards can be overwhelming tasks. Tackling them in smaller chunks not only makes them more manageable, but more enjoyable. Try writing out several cards each evening, rather than trying to do them all at once. Do your gift-buying online and avoid the annual mall death march through toy stores, factory outlets and discount palaces.

- Guard your sleep. Stress management and overall health demand adequate sleep and should top your priority list. The best way to ensure proper rest is to set regular bedtimes. Avoid or cut down on caffeine, alcohol and tobacco; all disrupt sleeping patterns, making it difficult to drift off or stay there. Eating too much food close to bedtime adversely affects slumber as well.

- Set reasonable goals over the holidays. If you want to shed fat, the holidays may not be the best time to do it. There are just too many tempting goodies around. In fact, it may be unreasonable to expect to lose any weight during the holidays. Maintaining your present weight, or only gaining two or three pounds instead of seven pounds or more, is a more sensible goal.

- Cancel the guilt trips. If, after all of your planning and commitment, you do overindulge, try not to feel guilty. Guilt only weakens your resolve to maintain healthy habits. Besides, guilt can spoil the fun of your holiday celebrations, and this is a time of year to be merry. Even if you do veer off your program, don't let that be your downfall. See the bigger picture, without obsessing over every little deviation from your plan. Simply do the next healthy thing for yourself: exercise, have a nutritious meal, or do some relaxation exercises.

- Be of good cheer. Send a contribution to someone in need, volunteer at a shelter, or contribute to a charity like Toys for Tots. Take a few moments of each day to simply say thank you for what you have. Release anger, bitterness and resentment. Be like a kid again in how you view the holidays; it will help you live with more wonder and enthusiasm. And finally, hold each day sacred. The present is the greatest gift of all.

If you take just a few pieces of my advice, I doubt if you'll have even one vision of a sugar plum or be tempted to sneak a nibble of the carolers' figgy pudding.

Review

- Pre-diet prior to the holidays. That way, you'll come into the season weighing less. Should you gain weight over the holidays, it won't be such a big deal.

- Eat strategically at parties and holiday gatherings so you don't go overboard.

- Fill up on fiber-rich foods to keep from overeating.

- Keep track of what you eat during the holidays by writing it down.

- Don't neglect exercise.

- Use stress-reducing techniques during the holidays.

- Remember the real reason behind the season.

LEAN 17: The 17 Most Fattening Holiday Foods and How to Downsize Them

Here are 17 holiday favorites from around the world. Note how they stack up calorie-wise and what you can do to soften the blow.

Food	Calories per Serving	The Leaner Eat
1. 8-ounce cheese ball	729	Opt for reduced-calorie cheese as an appetizer.
2. Eggnog (9 ounces)	343	Make your own low-fat version with egg substitute, evaporated skim milk, rum extract and some Truvia for sweetness.
3. Dinner roll	84 to 201	Serve whole wheat rolls or no bread at all.
4. Cranberry sauce (½ cup)	223	Serve reduced-sugar cranberry sauce and save around 150 calories.

(continued)

Food	Calories per Serving	The Leaner Eat
5. Candied yams (1 cup)	420	Mash sweet potatoes with a little orange juice; skip the sugar and marshmallows.
6. Mashed potatoes and gravy, large helping	240	Mash the potatoes with 2 parts potatoes and 1 part mashed parsnips, carrots, or cauliflower to reduce the calories. Use a little evaporated skim milk and forgo the butter. Skip or go easy on the gravy.
7. Potato pancakes (latkes), 2 pancakes	400	Use extra-virgin olive oil instead of higher-fat kinds such as corn oil, and toss out the egg yolks.
8. Creamed corn (1 cup)	184	Enjoy regular cooked corn kernels instead.
9. Traditional stuffing, large serving	640	Try wild rice as stuffing instead, and bake it separately in a covered casserole. Cooked inside the turkey, the stuffing absorbs too much fat from the meat.
10. Roasted goose	519	Stick with roasted turkey.
11. Prime rib	569 to 854, depending on the size of the slab	Control your portion size!
12. Roast pork with pineapple	466	Roast a pork loin in the oven by removing the skin, draining the fat, and adding broth, fruit, or bitter orange or orange juice instead of oil to keep it moist. Serve with pineapple canned in its own juice.

Food	Calories per Serving	The Leaner Eat
13. Tamales, 3	459	Rather than using lard or shortening, make the tamales with a healthier vegetable oil, such as olive or canola. You can also save fat and calories by making them vegetarian with a Mexican cheese or Monterey Jack and adding a green chile (jalapeño or Anaheim, for example) for an extra kick.
14. Lasagna, beef, 1 piece	377	Prepare vegetable lasagna and enjoy one piece instead of two. Or make lasagna the American way with lean ground beef, part-skim mozzarella and low-fat ricotta cheese and skip the cream.
15. Pecan pie, 1 slice (⅛ of the 9" diameter pie)	503	Pumpkin pie is a better bet. Some weigh in at only 150 calories a slice.
16. Apple pie, 1 slice (⅛ of the 9" diameter pie)	411	Go for pumpkin pie instead.
17. Christmas cookies	200	It's okay if you eat one, but who can stop at one?

MISTER MD, CAN YOU PLEASE TELL ME ?

I love the holidays, but I dread them, too, because when I start eating sweets, I can't stop. Why?

Sweet foods really do make you hungry. The more sweets you eat (no matter what kind), the more you crave them. Why? When you eat sugary stuff, your blood sugar (glucose) surges. Insulin then works hard to bring it down, and fast. But the plummet in blood glucose then increases your appetite. This may be why, after you eat sweets, you want more and more. Sweets also increase the feel-good brain chemical serotonin.

You've just got to cut back or avoid them altogether, and the cravings will ease up and may even disappear. Put off going grocery shopping during the holidays. The fattening stuff in your fridge will disappear first. After a few days, the cookies, ice cream and pecan pie are history. All that's left are the raw vegetables. This can force you to eat a healthy diet. If you procrastinate long enough before going grocery shopping, you might have to end up eating a raw beet. My point is: out of sight, out of mind. If holiday treats are calling your name, keep them out of earshot—which means out of your house.

GET SKINNY SHORTCUT

No Sweets

from your sweetie. Candy may be dandy for romance, but it can mean love handles in a hurry. Just about everyone likes candy on Valentine's Day, but most people are not aware of its calories. Most small pieces of chocolate—those about one ounce or so—contain about 150 calories each. It's not uncommon for a box of candy to contain 10,000 calories or more. If you eat the whole box, those excess calories can pile up faster than empty candy wrappers. And as far as timing goes, Valentine's Day is not calendar friendly, either. Most people are still trying to get rid of the excess pounds they put on during Christmas and New Year's. And before that came all of the Halloween candy. Ask your sweetie to romance you with flowers, perfume or a special spa day.

12

The 17 Day Diet on the Road

·····················

I once had a patient—I'll call her Tina—who flew occasionally. She was about 5'9" and weighed 155—not too bad for her height.

Then she accepted a job that immediately put her on a lot of airplanes. Tina liked to travel. But, while away from home, she wasn't exercising or eating as she knew she should be, and the end result was that she gained five pounds the first year. Didn't seem like much. But the next year she did the same; and the next. Tina gained an average of five pounds a year for five years. One look in the mirror told her even more graphically than her scales that she had an "excess baggage" problem.

Tina wasn't about to quit her job, but she was determined to lose that extra 25 pounds. She succeeded. And she kept it off. Not only did she feel better, but the mirror told her that she looked better, too. And according to the latest medical statistics, she should live longer as well. The only downside was that she had to buy all new clothes!

For Tina, losing that weight required a long-term commitment and a lot of determination. But she did it, even though she continues flying

239

100,000 miles a year and dealing with all the stuff that goes along with that level of travel.

If you're a "road warrior" like Tina, this chapter is for you. I've got some advice that I'm convinced will work for you as you take off weight while occupying the friendly skies, and elsewhere on your travels.

At the Airport

Let's be honest: most airport eateries aren't noted for the variety or quality of their offerings. Airports are filled with high-fat, high-sugar snacks. If I must chew on something, I stroll right past the kiosks selling junk food and look for places where I can buy fruit, low-fat yogurt or a salad.

Carefully examine the menus in airport restaurants. You can usually find a low-fat or low-calorie selection. If you have to grab airport food, look for a way to bulk up your fiber intake with things like fresh fruit (especially berries), salads, whole grains and vegetable soups.

What if you can't find anything that qualifies as "healthful?" Sometimes I simply go hungry a while longer. If I must order a less-than-healthful item, I eat only a small portion of it. (Be warned: this tactic requires extraordinary willpower.)

Be active. Avoid the moving walkway. Unless you're absolutely going to miss a connecting flight, walk briskly to your next gate using your own two feet without the mechanical help.

Walk the concourse. If you have time between connecting flights, start walking around at a comfortably fast pace. Sure, I know you might be tired after a long flight and don't want to trudge through the airport, pulling your carry-on through throngs of other passengers. But trust me, a little walk will rejuvenate you and prevent travel pounds from piling on. Try to get in at least 10 to 20 minutes of brisk walking.

On the Plane

Airline food is almost universally considered a bad dining experience. We've all seen those UFOs (unidentified fried objects) and had that ubiquitous chicken breast which has circumnavigated the globe many times by now. If you're on a flight that offers a meal service (or you're fortunate enough to have upgraded to a class that provides an actual meal), make the same choices you would in a restaurant. Choose the low-calorie, low-fat, healthful selections, and eat sparingly of those carb-rich items like rolls and desserts that aren't very healthful. Also, use only half the salad dressing you're given, and don't put butter on the roll. Ask if you can have some fresh fruit as a substitute for dessert. Little things add up fast.

Try to eat like you would at home. So if you don't tend to polish off a three-course meal with a giant hot fudge sundae at home, don't eat one on the plane. I guarantee it's not going to be the best hot fudge sundae you've ever had, so why blow it on something mediocre?

Don't drink too many calories. When the beverage cart rolls your way, ask for water, tomato juice or a calorie-free diet drink. Just say no to alcohol and beverages with caffeine because they contribute to dehydration. The snacks-for-purchase on flights aren't the greatest, so pass those up too. I suggest bringing your own healthy stuff to snack on: fresh fruits, cut-up veggies or one of my Power Cookies.

On long flights, move around from time to time. I don't mean roam the aisle and get in the flight attendants' way. Just stand up every half-hour or so and stretch your legs, arms and other muscles.

This doesn't just burn a few calories; it may help prevent deep-vein thrombosis (DVT), a serious medical complication of long flights. If your legs are immobile for long periods, blood can gather in them and form a clot in the veins found in the muscles. If the clot then travels to the heart, lungs or brain, it can be fatal. You're more at risk of a deep-vein thrombosis if you're elderly or obese, have a condition such as cancer or another acute medical illness, have undergone surgery, or are pregnant, on birth control pills, or on hormone replacement therapy.

There are other preventive measures you can take if you're at risk. A 20- to 30-minute brisk walk around the terminal building will keep your circulation going over several hours. Stay hydrated, too. Alcohol dehydrates you and makes you less mobile, increasing the risk of blood clots. Lots of airlines now offer exercise routines which you can do in your seat.

Traveling by Car

Don't forget your cooler, and pack your own meals, including low-fat snacks. Choose 98 percent fat-free lunch meats, fresh fruits and vegetables and water. Enjoy the trip by stopping at rest areas instead of fast-food chains. When eating from fast-food chains, choose wisely from the menu. Skip the French fries and mayonnaise. Go for the salads.

Food at the Hotel

Arriving at your hotel late in the evening after a long day of travel can make room service or a late-night restaurant seem very, very appealing. Don't give in! You may be hungry, but skip the meal. Avoid late-night eating. Eating heavy foods shortly before going to bed is one of the worst things you can do to your waistline.

If you must have something to eat, many hotels place a basket of apples at the front desk. Pick up one or two when you check in, and eat them before bedtime.

Sticking to a healthy nutritional regime can be a challenge when you're away from home. No matter where you go, much of your enjoyment will likely include great eats in different assignment destinations. Fortunately, there are ways to enjoy the local fare without the anxiety that can come from overeating.

Go online and research restaurants in a given community to determine which ones offer healthy choices. This exercise should be easy to carry out since many establishments pride themselves on their specialties, from fresh seafood, to down-home barbecue, to ethnic dishes. If you're heading to a major tourist town, look for guidebooks listing eateries according to cuisine type, as well as price range.

On a notepad, make a list of your leading picks in the following categories: best breakfasts, top lunch spots, and healthy restaurants for dinner. Then, tuck it into your purse, briefcase or glove box to keep it handy, so you'll have flexibility and enough choices for each category. When composing your list, skip all-you-can-eat places.

Start Your Day Healthy

If you begin your day with smart choices, chances are, you'll stick with the same mindset throughout the day. Cereal with low-fat or skim milk, fruit, yogurt, juice, bagels and the like are excellent choices. If you're staying in a hotel that offers complimentary breakfast or a free buffet, steer clear or limit your intake of greasy or fried items. Have regular, light meals throughout the day to keep your energy level up and calorie count in check. Of course, it's equally important to stay hydrated. Keep bottles of water on hand to prevent thirst and to curb hunger.

LEAN 17: 17 Packable, Travel-Worthy Snacks

1. 4 oz. applesauce cups (unsweetened)
2. Fat-free pudding snack cups
3. 4 oz. fruit cups, packed in fruit juice
4. Apple or pear
5. Lean granola
6. My Power Cookie
7. Cut-up raw veggies: carrots, celery, sugar snap peas, pepper or cucumber strips
8. Baby carrots
9. Single-serve box of high-fiber cereal
10. String cheese
11. One boiled egg
12. Small bag of fat-free popcorn
13. Small bag of grapes
14. Healthy sandwich with veggies
15. Beef or turkey jerky
16. Orange
17. Edamame

Exercising on the Road

Book a hotel with an exercise room, preferably one that's open twenty-four hours a day. This has become a "must have" for me. These days, the only way I'll stay in a hotel that doesn't offer exercise facilities is if I'm forced into it (for example, if I have to stay at a specific hotel in connection with a medical convention or meeting I'm attending).

If the hotel doesn't have fitness equipment, it may be affiliated with a local gym where you can get a one-day pass for a small fee. Once you get there, try a new class and a new instructor. You might be surprised at how fun it can be to do something different in another city. You might be able to find yoga, indoor cycling or step classes.

Spend a minimum of thirty minutes a day (or night) on the treadmill or stationary bike. You'll be surprised how good you feel at the end of your exercise time. You'll be more clear-headed and energetic for your business meetings, too.

I like to exercise in the morning. That way, I get it over with. At the end of a travel day there are too many variables that may get in the way. Besides, if you work out in the morning, you'll perform better all day.

Be creative. Most hotel rooms have enough floor space to allow you to turn your room into a mini-gym. Pack workout DVDs or jump ropes. Stack phone books for a step workout performed to a favorite exercise video.

Bring elastic exercise bands. Learn basic exercises by asking for help from a body-sculpting group exercise instructor or a personal trainer before you leave town. Practice so you can do the exercises proficiently while traveling. When you're back home, the bands will come in handy when you want to work out in your house or you can't make it to a health club.

But don't forget bodyweight exercises like pushups, squats with some luggage in hand to add extra resistance and overhead presses with the phone book. Sit-ups, with or without luggage resting on your chest, and crunches help round out any on-the-road fitness program. If you travel light, tune into exercise shows on television and join right in.

Mix business and pleasure. Go dancing at a local club. It's an easy way to burn calories and check out the local scene.

And don't forget your bathing suit. If the hotel has an on-site pool, swimming laps is a great way to work up a sweat (yes, you sweat while you swim) and wash away the day's stress.

Another trick I like is to ask for a room on the second floor or higher, so you can use the stairs in the hotel for a great workout. Mark off 17 minutes on your watch. Walk down the hall of the hotel to the stairs. Walk up a floor, then down the hallway of that floor. Go up another floor and walk that hallway. Continue in this manner for 8½ minutes; then repeat the "course" down and back to your room. Just make sure you get back to the right floor, and the right room. I've made that mistake before. It's not a pretty picture, trying to get in a room that's not yours.

Also, I bypass the elevator even if I'm carrying luggage and my room is located on the 12th floor. It's amazing how much cardiovascular benefit you can get from using the stairs instead of the elevator as you come and go. Sometimes, taking the stairs will get you to your room faster than the elevator will.

If stairs aren't your thing, consider the outdoors. How about seeing sights by walking, hiking or riding a rented bike? When renting bikes, rent helmets as well. Ask the local bike shop about the best and safest routes and for descriptions of the terrain (flat or hilly). Walking is a wonderful way to combine exploring a new place with maintaining fitness. It's my favorite travel workout because it lets me take in the local sights, smells and sounds. Wear supportive and comfortable shoes. Ask the hotel concierge for suggestions. Walking to your destination can also decrease your taxi fares.

Whew. I think I just burned 1,000 calories writing about all that.

So many people tell me they can't stay fit while traveling, but I don't buy it—that just means they don't want it badly enough. Good planning helps you fit fitness into your travel plans.

Review

- Make healthy choices at airports or on planes.

- Use the airport as a "gym" if you have time. Walk the concourse for exercise.

- Choose wisely at hotels, and when dining out.

- Start your day healthy with a nutritious breakfast and exercise.

- Book a hotel with a fitness center, or turn your hotel room into a gym.

- Handle vacations by keeping up your exercise program, planning for special dietary needs, focusing on non-food aspects of the vacation and making healthy choices.

How to Handle Vacations

"Would you like soup and salad to go with your meal?"

"What would you like for dessert?"

"Where should we eat today?"

"Let's hit the midnight buffet."

Recently, I was bombarded with these questions while on vacation. I was being offered 12-course meals, all-you-can-eat breakfast and lunch buffets and a grill that was open 24 hours a day.

But after days and days of enjoying delicious foods, I realized that vacations do not mean diet disaster. Vacations mean enjoying yourself while maintaining your weight. Yes, they present additional challenges when you are trying to lose weight and maintain an exercise program. An example I hear over and over again from people is: "I love going on cruises, but every time I do, I end up triggering myself to fall off my program for the rest of the year."

In cases like this, what should you do? I'd never suggest that you stop going on cruises or all-inclusive vacations, or to other destinations where food is so prevalent. But I might propose that you look for ways to be more active on one of these vacations, or plan to make healthier food choices or replace one of your yearly vacations with another type of vacation that is more active.

Vacations are not incompatible with watching your diet. They can always fit right into your lifestyle, and you don't have to feel burdened to overeat every time you go out of town or enjoy a holiday. There are always alternatives. Here are some practical suggestions to help you through vacations without undoing all the hard work you have put into losing weight:

- Decide on your goal over the vacation. Do you want to maintain your current weight or continue to keep losing weight? For weight loss, you'll have to monitor your calorie intake; if maintaining your weight is your goal, then you can adjust your calories upward slightly.

- If you have special dietary needs, plan accordingly. Some cruise lines, for example, offer heart-healthy meals low in fat and sodium and allow special orders.

- Focus on the other enjoyable aspects of the vacation, rather than the food—the locale, the sightseeing and the activities.

- Make healthy food choices as much as possible, with an emphasis on fruits, vegetables, whole grains and lean proteins. To keep your hunger in check, lean towards high-fiber foods and foods with a high water content, such as raw or steamed whole vegetables and fruits. A sensible approach can help you avoid overeating.

- Ask for special requests for food that may not be on the menu. Many resorts offer these types of dietary accommodations.

- Keep an eye on your serving sizes and always practice portion control.

(continued)

How to Handle Vacations—*continued*

- Join the walking, aerobics and dancing programs when you're on a cruise or resort, and use the exercise equipment in the gym. Take the most active shore excursions, or visit ports of call on your own and use guidebooks to create your own walking tour.

- Sightseeing activities get the muscles moving, but choose a tour that allows you opportunities to exercise. For example, time on your own in a city means you can jog or take a vigorous walk to attractions and shops. Ask whether the lodgings on a tour have lap pools or exercise rooms. If you happen to splurge, get back on course right away, whether this means taking a short walk or eating one healthy meal. Congratulate yourself for getting back on your program and acting in a healthy manner. After doing this a few times, you'll develop a positive mindset and begin to believe you can accomplish whatever it is you want.

13

Shift Work on the 17 Day Diet

I'm sure you've heard the song "9 to 5." It has catchy lyrics, but they don't describe the real-life experience of about 15 million Americans. That's how many shift workers—on duty evenings, nights, or on some rotating or otherwise irregular schedule—the U.S. Bureau of Labor Statistics estimates are in the workforce. And you may be one of them. Occupations affected include: the military, food services, transportation, manufacturing and industry, police, firefighters and security personnel, and health-care providers.

Unlike nocturnal animals such as owls and mice, most humans have some trouble adjusting to this strange lifestyle of working at night and sleeping in the day. This is because shift work, including night work, disrupts the body's "circadian rhythm"—the internal clock that governs eating, sleeping, body temperature and other regular biological processes, all hardwired and regulated to the rising and setting of the sun.

As it turns out, messing around with that clock can have some serious consequences for your weight. Shift workers have a higher prevalence of being overweight—a fact substantiated by research. There are four main reasons why.

First, regular eating and exercise habits are tough to maintain on shift work. You can get bored easily, so you tend to nibble on junk food in response. According to a study by the New York Obesity Research Center and published in *Nutrition* in 2000, late-shift workers gained an average of 9.5 pounds during their late-shift tenure, while their day-shift counterparts gained only 2 pounds.

Second, there's a hormonal issue. When you sleep and eat at irregular times, your metabolism gets thrown out of whack. At night, during sleep, your body's insulin-making processes naturally go into hibernation. You're not eating, so the body doesn't require much insulin to process glucose from food. But if you eat on your night shift, there's not much insulin action so your body drives nutrients toward fat accumulation this late in the day.

Third, digestive problems are at fault. Shift workers have two to three times as many digestive problems as their peers on the day shift. During nighttime, your digestive system shuts down and doesn't secrete the normal enzymes. Plus, your metabolism slows down in the evening. Many shift workers report diarrhea or constipation, gastric and peptic ulcers, gastritis, nausea and weight gain.

Finally, there are sleep problems. Shift workers are among the most sleep-deprived segments of our population. It's tough to sleep soundly during the day, when your body clock is screaming for you to be up and at it. Also, sleep deprivation drives down leptin, a hormone produced in fat cells that tells your brain when you're full. At the same time, your substandard snoozing causes a rise in ghrelin, a hormone that makes you feel like you haven't eaten since two Mondays ago. Numerous studies showed that those who sleep less than eight hours a night have lower levels of leptin, higher levels of ghrelin and more body fat than the long-slumbering subjects. Chronic sleep deprivation can thus drastically increase your risk of gaining weight.

The weird hours you have as a shift worker have a bunch of nutritional land mines—so here are some ways to avoid diet traps, stay true to the 17 Day Diet, keep your body in top form and still get your job done.

Avoid Junk Food

One of the things you can do to improve your energy and overall health is to eat a healthy diet, rich in vitamins and minerals. Those chocolate bars and packets of crisps in the vending machines at work may be tempting, but they're probably doing you more harm than good, reducing your energy levels and stamina even further. Doughnuts and cakes may give you an instant "buzz," but the downside is that you'll crash, and large amounts of refined sugar can lead to extreme mood swings.

The same goes for drinks. Cut down on the cans of Coke and other fizzy drinks (even the "diet" variety) and avoid beverages with caffeine because you'll find it harder to sleep when you get home. Instead, go for water. It's important to keep hydrated, since dehydration can lead to headaches and fatigue.

On night shift, eat small, light meals, with lots of raw salads, fruit and veggies, as recommended on the 17 Day Diet. These will give you energy but won't make you sleepy.

Sometimes shifts are long, so if you take sandwiches, make them whole grain bread. Try gluten-free bread. The older you get, the more difficult gluten is to digest and it can block the bowel. A healthy bowel that is moving will give you more energy.

Follow My Sample Shift Menus

Let's put these suggestions in concrete form. All Cycles of the 17 Day Diet are adaptable to shift work. It just takes a little bit of planning. If possible, take meals at approximately the same time each day, either midday or early evening, irrespective of whether you are on night shift. Follow the guidelines that follow, and you'll get in better sync, lose weight and be more alert.

Sample Shift Menu—Afternoon Shift
(Start time between 2:00 pm and 4:00 pm;
finish time between 10:00 pm and midnight)

Generally, if you work an afternoon shift, it's best to have your main meal (dinner) in the middle of the day rather than in the middle of your shift. You'll burn off your food better and stay more alert on your shift.

Here are some meal-planning suggestions for each Cycle.

Time of Day/Meal	Accelerate Cycle	Activate Cycle	Achieve Cycle	Arrive Cycle
8:00 to 10:00 a.m./ Breakfast	2 scrambled eggs, fresh fruit, 6 oz. yogurt	½ cup oatmeal or grits, cooked; 4 egg whites, scrambled; fresh fruit	1 cup cereal, high-fiber (e.g. Bran Buds or Fiber One); 1 cup (8 oz.) skim, 1% or soy milk or other dairy substitute; fresh fruit	Stick to whole grains and protein.
1:00 to 2:00 p.m. Dinner (before shift)	Grilled chicken breast with liberal amounts of any veg-etables, steamed or raw; fresh fruit	Pork sirloin chops, broiled or grilled; steamed veggies; ½ cup cooked corn; 6 oz. yogurt or other probiotic serving; fresh fruit	Grilled chicken; steamed vegetables such as asparagus, wax beans, broccoli or cauliflower; fresh fruit	Focus on protein-rich foods; they keep you alert.
7:00 to 8:00 p.m. Lunch at work break	Tuna tossed with 1 tablespoon olive oil and a tablespoon of vinegar, served over a generous bed of lettuce; 6 oz. yogurt or other probiotic serving to help with digestion	Shrimp salad: Cooked shrimp, 3 tablespoons chopped onion, generous bed of lettuce leaves, 1 tomato (large) and 1 tablespoon olive oil; 6 oz. yogurt or other probiotic serving to help with digestion	Pita sandwich: 1 whole wheat pita filled with chopped lettuce and tomato; 2 tablespoons crumbled fat-free feta cheese; 1 table-spoon Italian salad dressing; 10 baby carrots; 6 oz. yogurt or other probiotic serving to help with digestion	Continue focusing on protein-rich foods. Munch on fresh fruit and vege-tables. Don't overload yourself on carbs. Be sure to include probiotic foods to help with diges-tion

Time of Day/Meal	Accelerate Cycle	Activate Cycle	Achieve Cycle	Arrive Cycle
After work/ before bedtime	Have some fresh fruit.	Have a carb or two. Bananas are a good choice because they help with sleep.	Have a carb or two. Bananas are a good choice because they help with sleep.	Have a carb or two. Bananas are a good choice because they help with sleep.

Sample Shift Menu—Night Shift
(midnight to 8:00 a.m.)

Generally, night shift workers should snack lightly during their shift, eat a moderate breakfast and have dinner before their shift starts.

Here's a look at how to plan your diet.

Time of Day/Meal	Accelerate Cycle	Activate Cycle	Achieve Cycle	Arrive Cycle
When you wake up	2 scrambled eggs, fresh fruit, 6 oz. yogurt	½ cup oatmeal or grits, cooked; 4 egg whites, scrambled; fresh fruit	1 cup cereal, high-fiber (e.g. Bran Buds or Fiber One); 1 cup (8 oz.) skim, 1% or soy milk or other dairy substitute; fresh fruit	Egg-white omelet with spinach; one slice of whole wheat toast with jam; ½ cup fresh strawberries; tea, coffee or water
6:00 to 8:00 p.m./ Dinner (before shift)	Grilled chicken breast with liberal amounts of any vegetables, steamed or raw; fresh fruit	Pork sirloin chops, broiled or grilled; steamed veggies; ½ cup cooked corn	Grilled chicken; steamed vegetables such as asparagus, wax beans, broccoli or cauliflower; fresh fruit	Dinner: Green salad with sliced tomato, oil and vinegar dressing; ½ broiled chicken breast with lemon and herbs; ½ cup brown rice; steamed broccoli; fresh fruit cup; seltzer with lemon or water

(continued)

Time of Day/Meal	Accelerate Cycle	Activate Cycle	Achieve Cycle	Arrive Cycle
3:00 to 4:00 a.m. Lunch at work break	Tuna tossed with 1 tablespoon olive oil and a tablespoon of vinegar, served over a generous bed of lettuce; 6 oz. yogurt or other probiotic serving to help with digestion	Shrimp salad: Cooked shrimp, 3 tablespoons chopped onion, generous bed of lettuce leaves, 1 tomato (large), and 1 tablespoon olive oil; 6 oz. yogurt or other probiotic serving to help with digestion	Pita sandwich: 1 whole wheat pita filled with chopped lettuce and tomato; 2 tablespoons crumbled fat-free feta cheese; 1 tablespoon Italian salad dressing; 10 baby carrots; 6 oz. yogurt or other probiotic serving to help with digestion	Green salad with avocado and 4 oz. steamed salmon, oil and vinegar dressing. Iced tea, seltzer with lemon or water; 6 oz. yogurt or other probiotic serving to help with digestion
After shift, before sleep	Have some fresh fruit.	Have a carb or two. Bananas are a good choice because they help with sleep.	Have a carb or two. Bananas are a good choice because they help with sleep.	Have a carb or two. Bananas are a good choice because they help with sleep.

LEAN 17: 17 Foods that Keep You Alert

Most of the foods on the 17 Day Diet can help you stay more alert and are perfect for shift work. Choose more of the following foods if you're a shift worker.

Food	Alertness Factor
1. Beef, extra lean	High in iron, a mineral that improves memory, alertness and attention span.
2. Beets	Contain phenylalanine, an amino acid that helps relay signals from one brain cell to another.

Food	Alertness Factor
3. Blue-berries	Excellent source of antioxidants and anthocyanins, compounds thought to help protect brain cells from toxins, improve use of glucose in the brain and promote communication between brain cells.
4. Broccoli	Packed with antioxidants and phytonutrients that help protect brain tissue from toxins.
5. Carrots	High in beta carotene and other natural substances that help protect brain tissue from toxins.
6. Chicken	High in tyrosine, an amino acid required for the production of the alertness chemicals dopamine, epinephrine and norepinephrine. When your brain is producing these, you think and react more quickly, and feel more motivated, attentive and mentally energetic.
7. Citrus fruits	Contain vitamin C and other antioxidants that help maintain sharp memory and help brain cells resist damage.
8. Edamame	Contains phenylalanine, an amino acid that helps relay signals from one brain cell to another.
9. Eggs	High in the B vitamin choline, which helps with memory.
10. Egg whites	High in protein, which can improve alertness by increasing levels of norepinephrine, which helps keep your brain at its sharpest.
11. Hot chiles	Contain the fiery-tasting chemical capsaicin. Capsaicin stimulates circulation, aids digestion, opens your nasal passages and, even better, sends a feeling of euphoria straight to your brain.

(continued)

Food	Alertness Factor
12. Legumes	Provide glucose to fuel the brain, and the fiber they contain slows the absorption of glucose, helping to maintain stable levels of energy and support alertness and concentration over time.
13. Pork	Loaded with vitamin B$_1$, which protects myelin, a fatty substance that helps facilitate communication among cells.
14. Romaine lettuce	High in folate, a B vitamin important for memory and nerve cell health.
15. Spinach	Packed with iron, which is involved in memory, concentration, and mental functioning.
16. Tuna	Full of omega-3 fatty acids, which help build and maintain myelin.
17. Yogurt	A probiotic food that has been found in many studies to boost mental alertness. Yogurt and other probiotic foods are great foods for night shift work, since they help your digestion.

The Exercise Connection

Let's look on the bright side of the night shift: You get to go to the gym while almost everybody else is at work. Try picking a good time early in your "day." Even if you do only half your usual workout, you'll be moving your body, and you'll feel better. Seventeen minutes of exercise at least three times each week (though not just before bedtime) will help reduce stress and feelings of fatigue and increase your sense of well-being.

Be consistent with your training and add in some fun cross-training activities. You might have more time for outdoor bicycle rides, for example, with your night-shift schedule. As you catch up on your sleep, train longer and/or harder until you're back to your former training level.

Sleep Sense

Working when everyone else is asleep has advantages: less traffic for commuters, seeing newspapers being delivered, being around when the kids get home from school and maybe even a fatter paycheck. But getting enough rest isn't one of them.

Night-shift workers typically don't get the seven to eight hours of shuteye the vast majority of people need, and that's dangerous for your health, your weight and other people on the road when you're yawning behind the wheel.

Sleeping during the day tends to be less restful, too, so no wonder one in five night workers reports falling asleep on the job. I can't give you a surefire recipe for sound sleep during the day, but I have several techniques that should help. Even if each technique helps you sleep only a little better, altogether they may let you get the rest you deserve and need.

One key strategy is to maintain a somewhat constant schedule. Don't sleep from noon to 8:00 p.m. on Friday, then try sleeping nights on Saturday and Sunday, then switch back to day sleeping on Monday. Even if you alter your schedule somewhat, don't change too much. A study in the *New Zealand Journal of Psychology* advises a strategy called "anchor sleep," in which you include a three- to four-hour block of sleep time on non-shift-work days that coincides with your anticipated sleep time on shift-work days.

Sleep as soon as possible after the night shift. If you delay sleep after the night shift, your body will begin to warm up and prepare for the day's activity.

NOT THE USUAL 9 TO 5: Other Health Effects of Shift Work		
Conditions	*Reason*	*Strategies*
Cardio-vascular	Shift workers have more adverse lifestyle behaviors, such as higher tendency to smoke, not exercise, and eat junk food—all of which hurt the heart. In one study, 665 day workers were compared with 659 shift workers. The late-night workers had twice the risk of low HDL cholesterol, 40% higher risk of high triglycerides, and 19% higher risk of abdominal adiposity.	• Stop smoking • Exercise • Eat nutritiously
Breast Cancer	The risk may be associated with exposure to light at night. The hormone melatonin may play a role. Production of the hormone, which usually occurs during the "dark" period of a person's day, is disrupted by light exposure. The resulting dearth of melatonin may allow very small colonies of existing cancerous cells to flourish.	• Don't take melatonin, unless specifically recommended by a physician. While you'd think it would be helpful, it can throw a wrench into the smooth functioning of the circadian system and disrupt your biological clock.
Diabetes	Shift work can disrupt the body's insulin-making processes, potentially causing insulin resistance. With insulin resistance, the body doesn't use insulin properly. Glucose gets locked out of cells, and it clutters up the bloodstream.	• Have regular check-ups to monitor changes in blood sugar. • Avoid refined carbs such as sweets, white bread and baked goods. • Exercise regularly to help the body better regulate blood sugar.

Change your lights. You want the period while you're sleeping—whether you're a night-shift or daytime worker—to be as dark as possible. Consider blackout curtains, a sleep mask or anything else that reduces light. This is vital, since melatonin, the hormone of sleep which increases drowsiness, is suppressed by daylight even through closed eyelids. Light passes through your eyes and sets your brain's internal clock. You want to trick your brain into believing that day is night, and vice versa. No light? It must be night.

No matter what your shift, you may want to consider installing a low-wattage red bulb in the bathroom so that when you get up in the middle of your sleep cycle, it isn't disturbed by the shock of bright lights.

Sleep in a quiet part of the house, away from traffic noise and household activity. Tell family and friends about your schedule and ask them to call you only during waking hours. Give them a copy of your shift schedule.

Regulate your use of caffeine. Many of us toss back coffee to keep up energy at work. Not a good idea. It's tempting for night workers to use caffeine at the end of their shifts because it's when they're most sluggish, but that's only likely to continue to chip away at sleep quality.

Eat a banana or drink some warm milk before going to bed. Both these foods contain l-tryptophan, an amino acid known to be a natural sleep inducer. L-tryptophan releases serotonin, a sleep-inducing brain chemical.

Avoid alcohol prior to sleep. It is a diuretic and interferes with the quality of sleep.

Try an herbal tea prior to bedtime. Teas containing valerian root can be a safe, effective way to sleep when you really need to. As with any sleep aid, it should be used sparingly, however. Some people feel groggy upon awakening if they've taken valerian. (The best sleep aid is regular exercise.)

If you're a shift worker, you have to take extra care of yourself. It's worth your quality of life and livelihood to do so.

Review
....

- Shift workers suffer from obesity and other illnesses more often than people who work regular shifts.

- If you're a shift worker, avoid junk food. Have your main meal in the middle of the day if you work an afternoon shift, and have dinner just before your shift starts if you work the midnight shift.

- Populate your night with natural foods that keep you alert.

- Maintain a consistent exercise schedule.

- Practice good sleep health: keep your bedroom as dark as possible, sleep in a quiet part of your house, limit your use of caffeine and alcohol, and have a snack such as a banana and some warm milk prior to going to bed.

- Talk to your family doctor if you think you might be suffering from shift work disorder.

CHECKUP: Do You Have Shift Work Disorder?

The term shift work disorder, or SWD, may be new to you. But if you have a nontraditional work schedule, or work shifts, and are often tired on the job or have trouble sleeping, it's a condition you should learn more about.

Shift work disorder is a recognized medical condition that can be diagnosed and treated by a doctor. It occurs when your body's internal clock, or circadian rhythm, is out of sync with your work schedule.

Many people who work outside of the traditional 9-to-5 schedule need to be awake when the body's natural cycle calls for sleep. This disturbance of the circadian rhythm can lead to excessive sleepiness during waking hours or trouble sleeping during sleeping hours. If you're a shift worker, take the following quiz to see if you might have shift work disorder. Circle either "yes" or "no."

1. Do you feel tired no matter how much sleep you try to get? **Yes** **No**

2. Are you often less alert than you could be? **Yes** **No**

3. Do you have difficulty falling asleep or staying asleep? **Yes** **No**

4. Are you unaware of your total sleeping hours per day? **Yes** **No**

5. Have you been making more errors at work than usual due to lack of focus and general sense of fatigue? **Yes** **No**

6. Do you frequently suffer from heartburn or indigestion? **Yes** **No**

7. Do you experience occasional morning headaches? **Yes** **No**

8. Has your work, home or social life been negatively affected by sleeping problems? **Yes** **No**

9. Have you been experiencing unexplained weight gain? **Yes** **No**

10. Have you been experiencing irregular menstrual cycles? **Yes** **No**

11. Do you fall asleep while driving, in meetings, while reading a book, or while watching television? **Yes** **No**

Scoring: If you answered yes to three or more of these questions, you may be dealing with shift work disorder. Consult your doctor. He or she can help manage your symptoms. Only a change in shift work can resolve SWD, but there are some things you can do to try to cope with your symptoms, and they bear repeating:

- Avoid alcohol and other substances before bedtime.
- Get a full eight hours of sleep each day.
- Turning on bright lights may help diminish drowsiness when you need to be awake.
- Eliminate noise and light from your sleep area.
- Try to stick to your sleep and wake schedule, even on weekends.

14

The 17 Day Diet Recipes

. . . .

One healthy practice that will make a big difference in your weight loss is to cook your own food. Now before you start to panic, rest assured that you don't need to shout and jump and spin knives, make meals that look like a major work of art or get a degree from Cordon Bleu. You need some easy recipes—that's all. I can help you with that.

This batch of recipes is easy to follow and simple to prepare. There are no long lists of ingredients, complicated cooking methods or hard-to-understand directions. All the recipes are built around the foods you eat on the 17 Day Diet.

They're all low in fat and calories, made leaner and healthier by using cooking methods such as broiling, baking or lightly stir-frying. When the recipes do call for a bit of oil, it is always a healthy one like olive oil.

Some of the recipes make just one serving. If others in your family are following the 17 Day Diet, you can easily prepare these single-serve recipes in extra quantities. Other recipes yield multiple servings. Any leftovers can be refrigerated or frozen. That way, you can defrost and/or reheat in the microwave for a quick, healthy meal.

Once you get the hang of this way of cooking and eating, expect to lose your taste for greasy, sugary stuff. Why? Because tastes are learned. Just as you learned to like fattening, sugary or salty foods, your taste buds can be retrained to enjoy fresh, delicious and healthy dishes. For example, it's possible to retrain your taste buds by using herbs and spices. Salt-free seasoning blends are a good way to help yourself get out of the habit of sprinkling salt on everything. Your taste buds do adapt to what you eat.

I encourage you to get creative beyond these recipes. Most of us use the same 10 to 12 recipes most of the time. Why not try tweaking them to fit the 17 Day Diet? Here are some suggestions:

- **Dairy Products.** If a recipe calls for dairy products, you can always use low-fat and occasionally fat-free substitutions. For example, if a recipe uses one cup of regular sour cream, you can usually substitute with fat-free plain yogurt (Greek yogurt works great), or blended low-fat cottage cheese. Yogurt or silken tofu can be mixed with low-fat mayonnaise in dishes such as coleslaw, tuna and chicken salads.

- **Meats.** When selecting ground meats, look for those 90 percent fat free or higher. These are generally more expensive per pound, but you are getting more meat for your money because less fat is incorporated in the total product. If you cook ground meat, drain excess fat after browning it. Simply place a paper towel in a colander and pour the browned meat in so the towel can absorb the fat. If a recipe calls for a high-fat meat such as bacon, you can reduce the fat by 50 to 60 percent by using bacon bits to impart the flavor. Or try using Canadian bacon instead.

- **Bad Fats.** You can reduce or eliminate fats in recipes. For example, when sautéing or frying, simply coat nonstick pans with a spritz of vegetable oil cooking spray (0 calories) rather than using vegetable shortening or butter.

- **Spice it up.** Get in the habit of using high-flavor ingredients, like fresh herbs, zesty spices and seasonal fruit, rather than gobs of fat or oil, to invigorate dishes. Another tip: Buy an oil mister at a kitchen or housewares store (Misto is one popular brand). Simply pour oil, such as flaxseed or olive oil, into the spray bottle and then spray a fine mist of the oil over the pan or the food. This process drastically cuts the amount of oil that you use and reduces calories from fat.

- **Desserts.** Fruit makes a great dessert, but by itself may be boring to eat. Try dressing up a bowl of strawberries with a drizzle of sugar-free chocolate syrup. Also, you can easily redesign your favorite dessert recipes to yield less sugar, fat and calories by switching to lower-fat ingredients and learning how to cook with sweeteners such as Truvia.

- **Salt.** Are you watching your sodium intake? If so, start by using half the amount called for in the recipe. Continue to reduce the amount until you find the minimal amount needed to season the recipe. Or replace the salt with lemon or lime juice, flavored vinegar, fresh onion or garlic, onion or garlic powder, pepper, chili powder, ginger or other herb-only seasonings. Use low-sodium soy sauce or hot mustard sauce to replace regular soy sauce. Season food with spices and herbs as an alternative to adding salt.

Now—the 17 Day Diet recipes. Enjoy!

Dr. Mike's Power Cookie

Ingredients

⅓ cup unsweetened applesauce

2 tablespoons almond paste

1 tablespoon flaxseed oil

10 packets of Truvia

¼ cup agave nectar

1 large egg

½ teaspoon vanilla

¾ cup whole wheat flour

½ teaspoon baking soda

1 teaspoon cinnamon

½ teaspoon salt

¼ teaspoon black pepper

½ cup vanilla whey powder

2 cups oats

1 cup dried cherries

½ cup sliced almonds

Directions

Heat oven to 350 degrees. Beat together applesauce, almond paste, flaxseed oil, Truvia and agave nectar. Beat in egg and vanilla. Mix well. Add flour, baking soda, cinnamon, salt, pepper and whey powder. Beat thoroughly. Stir in oats, cherries and almonds. Mix well. Drop the batter by large tablespoons onto a cookie sheet that has been sprayed with vegetable cooking spray. Divide dough so that you have 18 cookies. Flatten each cookie with the back of the spoon. Bake 16 to 18 minutes or until brown. Remove from oven. Cool and store in a plastic container. Each cookie supplies 128 calories and can be enjoyed on the Activate, Achieve, and Arrive Cycles for breakfast or as a snack. Each cookie counts as 1 protein and 1 natural starch.

Kefir Smoothie

Ingredients

1 cup unsweetened kefir

1 cup frozen unsweetened berries

1 tablespoon sugar-free fruit jam
or 1 tablespoon agave nectar

1 tablespoon flaxseed oil

Directions

Place all ingredients in a blender and blend until smooth. Makes 1 large serving.

Yogurt Fruitshake

Ingredients

½ cup acidophilus milk

½ carton (3 oz.) sugar-free fruit-flavored yogurt

1 cup frozen unsweetened berries

Directions

Place all ingredients in a blender and blend until smooth. Makes 1 large serving.

Egg-White Veggie Frittata

Ingredients

4 egg whites, beaten

1 Roma tomato, chopped

Fresh spinach, handful

Salt and pepper, to taste

Directions

Coat a small frying plan with vegetable cooking spray. Add beaten egg whites. Stir in tomato and spinach. Cook on medium-low heat until egg whites are cooked through. Lift from pan with a spatula, and season lightly as desired. Makes 2 servings.

Spanish Omelet

Ingredients

1 egg

2 egg whites

⅛ teaspoon salt

⅛ teaspoon pepper

1 tablespoon olive oil

¼ cup diced tomato

2 tablespoons diced onion

2 tablespoons fat-free shredded cheddar cheese

Directions

In a medium bowl, whisk together egg, egg whites, salt and pepper. Heat a frying pan over medium-high heat. Add olive oil and swirl pan to coat bottom and sides. Add beaten eggs and tilt pan to spread mixture across entire pan bottom. Cook for about 30 seconds. With a spatula, gently lift sides of omelet and tilt pan to distribute more uncooked egg to the pan's surface. Once the egg begins to set, sprinkle tomato, onion, and cheddar cheese over one side of the omelet. Carefully fold the other side of the omelet over the fillings. Makes 1 serving.

Greek Egg Scramble

Ingredients

4 egg whites

¾ cup chopped red onions

¼ cup diced tomato

2 tablespoons reduced-fat feta cheese

⅛ teaspoon salt

⅛ teaspoon black pepper

Directions

In a medium bowl, whisk together all ingredients. Pour into a small frying pan that has been coated with vegetable cooking spray. Cook over medium-low heat until eggs are cooked through. Makes 1 serving.

Nicoise Salad

Ingredients

Cooked green beans, chilled
(½ cup to 1 cup)

2 chopped scallions

1 small tomato, sliced

Lettuce (the darker, the better)

1 3-oz. can light tuna

1 tablespoon olive oil

2 tablespoons balsamic vinegar

Directions

Place cooked green beans, scallions and tomato on a liberal bed of lettuce. Top with tuna. Drizzle with oil and vinegar and season lightly. Makes 1 serving.

Super Salad

Ingredients

Lettuce, any variety

Cucumbers

Onions

Tomatoes

Any salad vegetable from the 17 Day
Diet lists

2 hard-boiled eggs, chopped

2 tablespoons olive or flaxseed oil

4 tablespoons balsamic vinegar

Directions

Combine lettuce with salad veggies and hard-boiled eggs. Toss with oil and vinegar. Lightly season. Makes 1 serving.

Balsamic Artichoke

Ingredients

4 fresh artichokes

¼ cup balsamic vinegar

Fat-free salad dressing

Directions

Place artichokes in a large pot. Cover with water. Pour in vinegar. Cover and cook for approximately 1 hour on moderate heat, or until artichokes are tender, including the stems. Let cool. Serve with salad dressing for dipping. Makes 4 servings.

Spinach Salad

Ingredients

Baby spinach leaves (these taste less bitter than regular spinach leaves)

Assortment of salad veggies (onions, cucumbers, tomatoes, etc.)

2 tablespoons crumbled reduced-fat feta cheese

1 tablespoon olive or flaxseed oil

2 tablespoons balsamic vinegar

Directions

Place a large bed of spinach leaves on a plate. Top spinach with salad veggies and feta cheese. Drizzle with oil and balsamic vinegar. Season to taste. Makes 1 serving.

Taco Salad

Ingredients

1 pound lean ground turkey

1 envelope taco seasoning

Generous bed of lettuce

1 cup chopped tomatoes

2½ cups chopped onions

Salsa

⅓ cup shredded reduced-fat cheddar cheese

Directions

In a saucepan, brown ground turkey over moderate heat. Add the taco seasoning and cook according to package directions. Place generous servings of lettuce on 4 plates. Top with turkey mixture, tomatoes, onions, salsa and cheese. Makes 4 servings.

Village Salad

Ingredients

2 tomatoes, chopped

½ teaspoon sea salt

¼ cup chopped red onions

1 teaspoon dried oregano

1 tablespoon olive oil

2 tablespoons reduced-fat feta cheese

Directions

Combine tomatoes with sea salt; let sit for 5 minutes. Then mix tomato and salt together with the rest of the ingredients. Makes 1 serving.

Lettuce Wraps

Ingredients

1 baked chicken breast, diced

1 scallion, diced

½ cup chopped red grapes

2 tablespoons chopped celery

1 tablespoon olive oil

Salt and pepper to taste

2 to 3 Boston or iceberg lettuce leaves

Directions

Mix together all ingredients except lettuce leaves. Refrigerate until chilled. To serve, take 1 Boston or iceberg lettuce leaf at a time, and spoon a heaping tablespoon of the chicken mixture into the center. Wrap the lettuce around the filling. Makes 1 serving.

Spicy Yogurt Dip and Veggies

Ingredients

32 oz. fat-free plain yogurt

Garlic powder

Onion powder

Seasoned salt

Cut-up fresh veggies

Directions

Line a strainer with a coffee filter or white paper towel. Place the strainer over a bowl (this catches the liquid that will drain off the yogurt). Spoon the yogurt into the filter-lined strainer. Cover and refrigerate for 8 hours or overnight. This process yields about 16 oz. yogurt cheese (½ cup yogurt cheese = 1 probiotic serving). Season the cheese lightly with the seasonings suggested above, or add freshly chopped herbs such as parsley, rosemary or thyme. Use as dip for fresh vegetables.

Chicken-Vegetable Soup

Ingredients

1½ cups cabbage, chopped

1 large carrot, chopped

1 cup okra, sliced

1 large onion, chopped

2 large celery stalks with leaves, chopped

1 15 oz. can crushed tomatoes

1 14 oz. can fat-free chicken broth

1½ teaspoons salt

¼ teaspoon pepper

4 baked chicken breasts, diced into small chunks

Directions

Place all ingredients, except chicken, in a large pan and simmer for one hour or until vegetables are soft. Add chicken and heat thoroughly. Enjoy this soup for lunch or dinner. Makes 4 servings.

Marinated Vegetable Salad

Ingredients

4 cups raw vegetables
(green beans, cauliflower, Brussels sprouts, artichoke hearts, etc.)

Fat-free Italian dressing

Jarred roasted red peppers (without oil)

Directions

The night before, steam vegetables in at least 2 cups water until they're tender but still crisp. Place in a glass dish and pour dressing over veggies. Refrigerate overnight. Drain and serve on a bed of lettuce and top with red peppers. Makes 2 to 4 servings.

Eggplant Parmesan

Ingredients

1 large eggplant, peeled

4 egg whites

Fat-free Parmesan cheese

Garlic powder, to taste

1 cup low-carb marinara sauce

Directions

Preheat oven to 400 degrees. Cut eggplant into ¼-inch slices. In a shallow dish, beat egg whites and 4 tablespoons water until foamy. Dip eggplant slices into egg whites, then into Parmesan cheese, pressing cheese into eggplant. Place eggplant on prepared baking sheet that has been sprayed with vegetable spray and sprinkle with garlic powder. Spray vegetable cooking spray over eggplant slices. Bake 30 minutes, turning eggplant over after 20 minutes, until golden brown and cooked through. Cover with 1 cup marinara sauce. Bake for 20 minutes, or until eggplant is piping hot and sauce is bubbly. Makes 2 large servings.

Sesame Fish

Ingredients

1 pound tilapia

2 tablespoons olive oil

2 tablespoons rice vinegar

2 tablespoons lite soy sauce

1 teaspoon chopped garlic

2 tablespoons sesame seeds

Directions

Spray a broiler pan with vegetable oil spray. Place tilapia in pan. Whisk together olive oil, rice vinegar, soy sauce and garlic until well blended. Pour over fish. Sprinkle sesame seeds over fish. Broil at medium heat about eight inches away from heat for about 20 minutes or until fish flakes easily with a fork. Makes 4 servings.

Salmon Lemenato

Ingredients

2 pieces wild salmon

1 tablespoon olive oil

3 cloves fresh garlic, chopped

3 lemons

1 teaspoon dried oregano

Directions

Preheat oven to 350 degrees. Place salmon in a shallow glass dish that has been sprayed with vegetable cooking spray. Drizzle olive oil over salmon. Top with garlic. Squeeze the juice of the lemons over the salmon and sprinkle with oregano. Bake for 25 minutes. Makes 2 servings.

Oven Barbecued Chicken

Ingredients

4 skinless boneless chicken breasts

¾ cup reduced-sugar ketchup

2 tablespoons Worcestershire sauce

1 tablespoon agave nectar

1 teaspoon chili powder

Directions

Preheat oven to 350 degrees. Place chicken breasts in a baking pan that has been sprayed with vegetable cooking spray. Bake for 20 to 25 minutes. In the meantime, stir together ketchup, Worcestershire sauce, agave nectar and chili powder to make the barbecue sauce. Remove chicken breasts from oven and coat with sauce. Return to oven and bake for 10 more minutes. Makes 4 servings.

Turkey Black Bean Chili

Ingredients

1 pound lean ground turkey

2 cups black beans (for Cycles 2 and 3 only)

1 cup chopped onion

2 cups tomato sauce

1 tablespoon chili powder

1 teaspoon Kosher salt

½ teaspoon black pepper

Directions

In a saucepan, brown ground turkey over moderate heat. Add the remainder of the ingredients. Simmer for 20 minutes. Makes 4 servings.

Low-Carb Primavera Delight

Ingredients

1 spaghetti squash

2 cups chopped fresh broccoli

1 small onion, diced

2 diced garlic cloves

1 tablespoon olive oil

Marinara sauce

Directions

Spaghetti squash is a great substitute for pasta. To prepare it, cut it in half (lengthwise). Scoop out the seeds and pulp as you would with any squash or pumpkin. Place it in a glass baking dish with about ½ inch of water, rind side up. Bake 40 to 45 minutes at 375 degrees. You can also microwave the squash for 8 to 10 minutes per half on high. Let the squash stand for a few minutes after baking or microwaving. Separate strands by running a fork through in the "from stem to stern" direction. Place strands in a separate bowl.

In a medium frying pan, sauté broccoli, onion, garlic and oil until vegetables are crisp tender. Add squash and heat thoroughly. Serve on plates and top with heated marinara sauce. Makes 4 servings.

15

Mister MD, Can You Please Tell Me More?

The **17 Day Diet** is simple, easy and doable, but still questions arise from time to time. Here are the questions I'm frequently asked, along with my answers. This information will help you.

Diet Issues

Q. I just need to lose those "last 10 pounds." How long should I stay on the diet?

A. You should lose those 10 pounds rapidly on Cycle 1, if you follow it to the letter. Or you may have to continue into Cycle 2. It all depends on your individual metabolism. Everyone is different and loses weight at different rates. If you'd like to accelerate your weight loss and get to that goal faster, increase your exercise time and intensity each day. Just hang in there, don't get discouraged, and you'll achieve your goal weight in no time.

Q. Can I switch some dinners to lunches, and lunches to dinners?

A. Yes, you may switch lunches with dinners. It is a good idea to eat lightly in the evening anyway. I recommend switching lunches and dinners if you are a shift worker, especially. If you switch, be sure not to eat carbs past 2:00 p.m.

Q. Is the 17 Day Diet safe for everyone?

A. The diet is designed for people in normal health. Anyone who goes on this diet should first get the approval of his or her physician. Do not follow this diet if you have type 1 diabetes or any serious medical disease, or if you are pregnant or nursing.

Q. I've gotten great results so far on Cycle 1. Can't I just stay on it?

A. Great job with your weight loss! That tells me you have a strong will for healthier habits and respect the gift of your health. Keep going! I don't advise staying on Cycle 1 more than 17 days, however. The diet is carefully designed to keep your metabolism charged up, to prevent plateaus, and to re-introduce foods gradually back into your life. It's best that you follow all three Cycles as described. Then, after 51 days, you get to return to Cycle 1 for continued weight loss.

Q. Can I drink fruit-flavored green tea on the diet?

A. Yes, as long as it is not sweetened with added sugar. Many green teas in the supermarket are flavored with a hint of natural fruit and no added sugar. These are very tasty and can be enjoyed hot or cold.

Q. When you say "liberal amounts" of a food, does that mean a huge piece of meat or second helpings of those foods?

A. No. It's important not to overload your stomach. Use my Hunger/ Fullness Meter to keep that from happening. Eat until satisfied, not to the point at which you feel like your stomach is going to explode.

Q. There is a lot of protein on the 17 Day Diet. Why?

A. Protein is the major component of all of your body's cells, and it's important to make sure you're getting enough. Recent research indicates that we may need more than previously thought. The recommended dietary allowance (RDA) for all adults is 0.37 grams of protein per pound of body weight, or about 15 percent of your daily calories. You may need more if you exercise, if you're dieting and as you age.

One dramatic study of 855 people found that those who ate just the RDA of protein had alarming bone losses compared to those who ate more than the RDA. Those who ate the least protein lost the most bone mass: 4 percent in four years. People who ate the most protein (about 20 percent of calories) lost less than 1.5 percent in four years, reported the *Journal of Bone and Mineral Research* in 2000.

Although the study was done on older men and women, the results may be important for all adults. When you're young, you need protein to build bone. After age 30, you need it to keep bone from being lost. Keeping bones strong is a life-long effort.

As for weight loss, take note: Research keeps proving that a protein-dense diet is essential for weight loss. It helps maximize fat loss while minimizing muscle loss. That's important because losing muscle slows your resting metabolic rate—the speed at which your body burns calories. That makes it harder to maintain a healthy weight and lose fat. By eating regularly from the foods on the 17 Day Diet lists, you'll get more than enough protein.

Q. I'm a vegetarian. Can I follow the 17 Day Diet?

A. Yes. If you're a "lacto-ovo-vegetarian," you limit your protein to dairy products and eggs. That means you'll obtain your protein from probiotics like yogurt, eggs, and beans and legumes (depending on which Cycle you're on). "Semi-vegetarians," who avoid red meat but eat fish or chicken, can easily follow the diet. "Vegans" avoid all animal proteins. If you're a vegan, you can still follow the diet. Simply use vegan meat substitutes at meals for protein and use a probiotic supplement in place of yogurt.

Q. I know that whole grains are really good for me, but I get bored with oatmeal and brown rice. What are some other ones I can try?

A. There are plenty of other choices. Look into some of the so-called ancient or alternative grains: amaranth (high in protein), kamut (a cousin of wheat), quinoa (a grain-like herb), spelt (a relative of wheat), triticale (a cross between rye and wheat), whole grain risotto (a delicious type of rice), barley (super-high in fiber) and bulgur (a delicious form of wheat). To find some of these more uncommon grains, you may need to try a big natural foods store or local ethnic food market. Many of these grains are unfamiliar to Americans but have been eaten in other parts of the world for thousands of years.

Q. Sometimes I can't eat all the food allowed on the 17 Day Diet. Will this interfere with my results?

A. No, not at all. The 17 Day Diet is very filling. For many people, it's a challenge to eat all those fruits and vegetables for the first time. If you can't eat all the food, don't worry about it. Just don't replace those foods with foods not on the diet.

Q. I overindulged all weekend. What do you suggest?

A. If you gained 3 to 5 pounds over the weekend, I advise that you go right back to Accelerate (Cycle 1) until you lose those pounds. After that, continue on with the other Cycles to reach your goal.

Nutrition Questions

Q. Is it better to choose organic foods?

A. These days, we need to find out where everything comes from and how it's been grown or raised. Is it organic, cage-free, free-range, or was it just grown in someone's backyard? We do need to reduce our exposure to toxins, or else they get stored in our bodies' fat cells. Scientists think this build-up of toxins may prevent weight loss. So buy organic whenever you can. Eating organic foods helps you naturally rid your body of toxins. Because some produce contains more pesticides than others, try to choose organic when shopping for these fruits and veggies: apples, nectarines, peaches, pears, strawberries, raspberries, cherries, imported grapes, bell peppers, celery, potatoes and spinach.

Q. What is your recommendation on taking a standard multivitamin?

A. I'm in favor of it. Taking vitamins and other supplements is important, but it can take quite a bit of time to pop everything you need. You may require a multiple vitamin and mineral, omega-3 fatty acids to reduce inflammation, calcium for bones and vitamin D.

Multivitamins can be especially helpful for anyone who doesn't eat a healthy diet or eat enough "good" foods to obtain the vitamins we need for sustained good health. Plus, as we age our bodies don't absorb certain vitamins, such as vitamin B12, as well as they once did. We also need more vitamin D and calcium, but those can be consumed in separate supplements.

If you feel a multivitamin is important to your health, bring a bottle of vitamins to your doctor to make sure the doses are safe (megadoses of some vitamins can be dangerous), and make sure that there are no potential interactions between the vitamin supplements and any prescription drugs you're taking.

Q. You recommend a sweetener called TruviA. What is it?

A. Truvia is derived from stevia, a plant found in South America and Asia. This means that it is neither a sugar nor a purely artificial sweetener, but is instead a "natural" zero-calorie sweetener. Truvia also contains erythritol, a kind of sugar alcohol found in fruits. As sugar substitutes go, Truvia and stevia are probably better than some lab-produced artificial sweeteners, which is why I recommend it. You can also cook and bake with Truvia. But like anything else, use it in moderation.

Q. Can I use other sugar substitutes on the 17 Day Diet?

A. Artificial sweeteners are found in many foods these days, such as reduced-sugar yogurt, which is one of the recommended probiotics on the 17 Day Diet. Clinically speaking, all sugar substitutes are testing safely; we just don't know much about their long-term health effects.

Six of the most common sugar substitutes currently available are aspartame (Equal), saccharine, acesulfame K, sucralose (Splenda), sugar alcohols and stevia (Truvia and Sweet Leaf). Aspartame, saccharine, acesulfame K, and sucralose are all chemical sugar substitutes that do provide some health benefits: They are lower in calories than regular sugar, and they do not raise blood sugar, particularly helpful for people with diabetes. Nor do these sweeteners promote tooth decay.

Sugar alcohols, such as mannitol and xylitol, are carbohydrates but not sugars, which makes them sugar-free sweeteners. Unlike artificial sweeteners, they can raise blood sugar, but because they are slowly absorbed from the intestinal tract, the rise in blood glucose and demand for insulin is minimal compared to eating pure sugar. They, too, are low calorie compared to natural sugar and do not promote tooth decay. Stevia is a newer artificial sweetener that is natural in the sense that it is not a chemical made in a lab. It is a natural extract from the stevia plant.

My advice is to go easy on sugar substitutes and learn to enjoy the natural sweetness of fresh fruits.

Q. I am trying to kick my sodium habit. Do you have any suggestions?

A. You might start by using a lite salt, such as Morton's Lite salt, to wean yourself off sodium. Start cooking with herbs and spices too, especially garlic and onion powder to season meat or vegetables.

When buying foods, purchase reduced-sodium versions. Buy and use the sodium-free marinades for chicken, beef, pork and seafood.

When buying and using canned vegetables and beans, rinse them under running water to remove up to 40 percent of the sodium.

The taste for salt is a learned habit. Just as you acquired a taste for salty foods, you can also become accustomed to less salt.

Q. I've been hearing more and more about the health benefits of coffee and tea. But they both have caffeine, right? Which has more?

A. The fact that coffee and tea are good for you isn't new. The first written records of coffee mention it as a medicine. Over the years, herbalists have thought it could treat head and muscle aches, asthma and fatigue. Early references to tea in China involve boiling raw, wild tea leaves in water to soothe respiratory infections.

You already know that the caffeine in your morning cup of coffee keeps you alert and active. Now the Harvard Nurses' Health Study, a long-term examination of the habits of more than 100,000 nurses, has shown that there is a decreased risk of developing type 2 diabetes among participants who regularly drink coffee (caffeinated or decaf). Coffee is terrifically high in antioxidants, along with minerals, such as potassium and magnesium and B vitamins. All of these nutrients might be the reason coffee guards against type 2 diabetes.

The good coffee news just keeps on coming: Research linked regular coffee consumption (three to four cups per day) to a decrease in the incidence of Parkinson's disease. Scientists have found that an extra espresso may even help stave off mental decline as you age, said a 2002 study in the *American Journal of Epidemiology*.

So grab a cup of coffee, sink into an oversized chair, and read on.

Q. If coffee and tea are so good for us, should I drink more?

A. Well, too much of any good thing becomes not such a good thing. How much you consume depends on your health and your caffeine tolerance. Most docs say three to four 8 oz. cups of caffeinated coffee or tea is the maximum that an individual should have daily.

Be aware that caffeine stimulates the central nervous and cardio-vascular systems and is a diuretic. Too much coffee or tea can result in elevated blood pressure, insomnia, nervousness or rapid, uncomfortable breathing. Also, tannins found in coffee and tea may decrease your ability to absorb iron, so drink them at least one hour before meals so you can digest the tannins before iron is released in your system.

Q. I keep hearing people knock high-fructose corn syrup. What is it exactly? And is it really bad for you?

A. High-fructose corn syrup (HFCS) is a potent sweetener made from corn starch. It's actually twice as sweet as sugar. Manufacturers began using it as a cheap sugar substitute in the 1970s when the price of sugar shot up. HFCS now accounts for 40 percent of the caloric sweeteners added to foods and drinks.

Americans down about 132 calories' worth of HFCS a day, mainly in sodas and fruit drinks. That's a lot. By simply slashing 132 calories daily, you can lose about 13 pounds a year without doing anything else.

But calories aren't the real concern with HFCS: It seems to make us pig out in two ways. First, when soda manufacturers switched from sugar to HFCS, they used the same quantity by volume, so sodas today are much sweeter than they were 30 years ago. Regular exposure to their intense sweetness can make you crave other sweets too.

Second, your body metabolizes HFCS differently. Unlike other sweeteners, HFCS doesn't produce a normal rise in insulin after a meal, which prevents the usual levels of a hormone called leptin that makes you feel full. Too little leptin, and you'll eat too much. From everything I've read, I recommend avoiding HFCS.

Q. I've heard over and over again that trans fat is bad for us. What I'm not sure of is what it is. And why is it bad?

A. Trans fat is formed when unsaturated oils are put through a chemical process called hydrogenation. This process solidifies the oils at room temperature: think margarine or vegetable shortening. Hard fat is necessary to achieve specific characteristics in certain foods. For example, without a hard fat, crackers would be soft, pie crusts would lose their flakiness and foods would go rancid more quickly.

Not all hard fats are trans fats though; some are saturated fats (the kind found in butter, cocoa butter, and palm and coconut oils). But several years ago, the food industry moved away from using saturated fat because of its association with increased LDL ("lousy" cholesterol) levels. In making this switch, the industry unknowingly created a fat that has turned out to be even worse for health: trans fat. In recent years, scientists have discovered that trans fatty acids not only raise LDL levels, they lower HDL ("good" cholesterol)—increasing your risk factors for heart disease. They also increase obesity.

Fortunately, fewer products are being manufactured with trans fats. If you're worried about whether a product contains trans fat, look on the ingredients label for the term "partially hydrogenated." Partially hydrogenated oil is trans fat.

Q. Are imitation seafood products good choices?

A. Imitation crab, shrimp, and other seafood (surimi) are usually made from Alaskan pollock, a whitefish. The skinless, boneless fish is ground up, mixed with binders, salt and other flavors, cooked and then shaped. This imitation shellfish is an excellent source of low-fat protein and is lower in cholesterol than true shellfish.

A disadvantage is that it can contain nearly 700 milligrams of sodium in a modest three-ounce portion. That's almost a third of the sodium limit recommended for a whole day and almost half of the limit recommended for people with sodium-sensitive high blood pressure.

Imitation seafood tastes pretty good. But if you don't like to eat ingredients that sound unnatural, stick to the real deal.

Q. Every year I resolve to eat healthier, and I do—for two weeks or a month. How can I keep from falling back into my old diet patterns every year?

A. First of all, keep making resolutions. Studies show that people who resolve to quit smoking, lose weight or start an exercise program are much more likely to succeed than people who don't.

Second, take action. Sitting around, thinking about change, and talking about it doesn't make a difference. What produces change is action. Here are some action-oriented behaviors known to work for weight loss and prevent relapse:

- Eat breakfast every morning and regular, planned meals throughout the day.

- Exercise regularly. This concept is really simple—move it AND lose it.

- Guzzle more aqua. Water will really fill you up and assist in fat-burning.

- Start a love affair with veggies. Supplement your meals with healthy salads and veggies and make your mom proud.

- Eat before going to parties or other food-centered gatherings.

- Plan get-togethers with friends that don't revolve around food.

- Reward yourself for progress (but not with food), and ask friends and family members to do the same.

- In short, set a goal or resolution, plan concrete steps that will take you there, anticipate and avoid pitfalls and reward yourself along the way.

Health Issues

Q. Just about everyone in my family is overweight. Is the deck stacked against me?

A. Yes, there is the genetic piece to consider. People who research obesity discovered the "blame-your-parents" factor. Their studies involved fat twins who were adopted by separate thin families. The twins remained heavy despite their slim surroundings. The study concluded that the ring around your middle, or at least some portion of it, comes from your parents, not just from what you eat when nobody is looking.

So yes, a family history of obesity may increase your odds of ending up overweight, but that just means you may have to work a little harder than those without such a history to achieve and maintain a healthy weight. You're not doomed. In fact, researchers in Great Britain found that exercising can reduce the genetic tendency toward obesity by 40 percent. Their findings were reported in *PLoS Medicine* in 2010. You can choose to adopt healthy habits. We inherit predispositions to certain problems, including obesity, but we also have the power to decide what to do about them.

Q. Does stress make people fat?

A. It appears there is some connection, and it's based on the theory of the "caveman paunch." It has to do with where fat settles in the body, and it goes something like this. Guys get beer bellies for the same reason women get thunder thighs: it's a product of evolution. Cavewomen laid down stores of fat in their thighs and breasts to cope with the demands of pregnancy in the wild.

In cavemen, flight-or-fight energy was stored as belly fat. When cavemen went beast-hunting and suddenly ended up being the hunted, their guts dispersed the fuel (fat) their muscles needed to high-tail it to safety. Since cavemen spent a lot of time fleeing, they never had much of a weight problem.

Nowadays, however, our predators are bosses, phone solicitors and issuers of credit cards. They are irritating, and it's hard to get away from them. A good idea is to lace up your sneakers and go for a brisk walk. It's like hunting beasts but without any weapons. Regular exercise, seriously, really does prevent stress fat, plus a lot of other things.

Q. I'm a smoker. I know I should quit. But I'm afraid I'll gain weight. What do you think?

A. Let me ask you some questions: Are you sacrificing what might help your health in the name of keeping off a few pounds? Where is your common sense? You might be surprised to learn that if you exercise while quitting smoking, you won't gain weight.

Kicking butt with exercise will help you kick your cigarette habit. An Austrian study found that after three months, 80 percent of smokers who did a cardio and strength-training workout three times a week while using a nicotine-replacement therapy of their choice (such as a patch, gum, inhaler or combination of them) had given up smoking; only 52 percent of those who used nicotine replacement alone were successful. Plus, unlike such tools as prescription medications, exercise has no negative side effects. Confer with your doctor and walk, cycle and jog your way to a smoke-free and strong, fit body.

Q. I'm 56, and I've recently been diagnosed with prediabetes. What kind of screening tests should I have, and what should I do to help make sure it doesn't progress to diabetes?

A. Prediabetes is when a person's blood glucose levels are higher than normal, but not high enough for a diabetes diagnosis. If you are prediabetic, you have a greatly increased risk of heart attack, stroke, cancer, kidney disease, blindness, nerve damage and other conditions.

Given your recent diagnosis of prediabetes, your doctor may recommend you check your blood sugar at home. Whether or not this is the case, there are several lab tests which are important for you to have run at regular intervals. The most important are the fasting blood glucose and the hemoglobin A1C (HgbAlC). This latter test indicates the average level of your blood sugar during the previous three months. A normal value for the HgbAlC is from 4 to 6 percent, and the goal for those with diabetes is to treat to below 7 percent. Whether you are treating your prediabetes with only lifestyle modifications such as diet, exercise and weight loss, or you are on medication, the HgbAlC should be checked at least twice a year, more often if your doctor recommends it.

There are several things you can do to help treat prediabetes and prevent the onset of type 2:

- **Eat a healthy diet and lose weight:** Losing only 5 percent to 7 percent of your current body weight can usually bring the blood sugar down to normal ranges.

- **Exercise:** Get at least 30 minutes of activity a day, five days a week. Fat blunts insulin's ability to lower blood sugar. With less fat on board, your blood sugar can normalize.

- **Treat high blood pressure and cholesterol:** If you have been told that you have either of these conditions, speak to your doctor on the best course of treatment to get them in check.

- **Quit smoking:** Diabetes is not the only reason to quit, as smoking contributes to many other health problems.

- **Educate yourself:** Education is key for prediabetes and type 2 diabetes management. Diabetes is a complex condition and needs close monitoring to help you remain as active and healthy as possible. Most insurance plans provide coverage for diabetes education programs, and they are very helpful in assisting newly diagnosed patients with diabetes management.

Q. What are the best foods for my joints?

A. If your joints hurt, they might be inflamed. But popping painkillers isn't the only way to stop the pain. You can eat your way to more comfort with a fresh, unprocessed diet, as I suggest on the 17 Day Diet. Try eating fish like sardines, wild salmon or cod at least twice per week. Include daily servings of whole grains and legumes, fruits (particularly berries) and vegetables—basically all the foods that are a part of the 17 Day Diet. These will give you the vitamins and minerals, omega-3 fatty acids and other nutrients you need to protect cells from inflammation.

Another common and generally safe remedy is glucosamine, available as a supplement. Many people get relief when they take it. Consult your doctor about whether to take, which kind to take, and how much.

Q. My HDL cholesterol is low. What can I do to raise it?

A. Weight control and regular physical activity are the most important steps you can take to raise your "good" HDL cholesterol. Higher HDL levels (60 mg/dl or above) are linked with lower risk of heart disease, while low HDL (40 mg/dl and below) is considered a major cardiovascular risk factor and is now being linked with greater risk of memory loss later in life. Low HDL levels are often associated with being overweight, especially if excess body fat is congregating at the waistline.

Studies suggest that overweight people who reach and maintain a healthier weight may raise low HDL levels anywhere from 5 to 20 percent. Daily moderate aerobic physical activity, such as walking or swimming, is also very effective at raising low HDL. Although some people assume a low-fat diet is beneficial, completely cutting out heart-healthy fat (such as olive oil or omega-3 fats) can hurt rather than help your efforts. In addition, avoid smoking, which is linked with lower HDL, and make sure that blood sugar is under control.

Genetics play a role in your HDL levels, and it's hard to change genetics. But with diet and exercise, you have two breakthrough tools to help you increase your HDL. Both are really the best medicine—and safe and cheap, too!

Q. Are there foods I can eat for better skin?

A. Yes. Foods rich in "beauty nutrients" can make your skin clearer, smoother and more radiant. Salmon is an excellent source of omega-3 fatty acids, which lubricate skin from within and prevent acne; kiwis and blueberries provide vitamin C, which helps prevent wrinkles; oysters are rich in zinc, crucial for collagen production; and sweet potatoes and tomatoes contain carotenoids, which may protect skin against damaging UV rays.

Q. Can people who are already overweight reduce their cancer risk if they lose weight?

A. Many adult cancers develop over a 10- to 20-year period or longer. Although researchers can't say for sure that losing weight will lower cancer risk, the evidence looks promising.

For example, two large studies of post-menopausal women found that those who lost weight after menopause reduced their risk of breast cancer substantially. That's important since reports estimate that overweight and obesity in the United States account for 14 percent of cancer deaths among men and 20 percent among women.

When overweight people lose weight, they may not be able to undo cancer-causing damage that's already done, but shedding excess fat can reduce elevated levels of insulin, insulin-related growth factors and certain hormones like estrogen. All these compounds are associated with the process of cancer development. Each loss or gain of excess body fat seems to change cancer risk.

Q. Is it true that sugar "feeds" cancer?

A. While all cells in our bodies use sugar (glucose) for fuel, research does suggest that cancer cells take up blood sugar more rapidly than healthy cells. In addition, high blood sugar stimulates increased levels of insulin in the body, which may promote the growth of cancer cells.

Although this may sound frightening, the answer is not to avoid all sugar-containing foods. The sugar in our bloodstream comes from all carbohydrate foods, including healthful vegetables, fruits, whole grains and low-fat dairy sources; some glucose is even produced within our bodies from protein.

For now our best answer is to keep blood sugar controlled with weight maintenance, regular exercise and a high-fiber diet. It's also important to avoid big loads of carbohydrate at once, particularly from refined grains like white bread or foods with added sugars. Hopefully, further research will provide more answers.

Food Allergies

Q. An allergist recently told me I suffer from lactose intolerance. What can be done about this, as I find it hard to face a life without dairy products?

A. Lactose intolerance is caused by a lack of one or more enzymes that digest lactose, the carbohydrate in milk. Symptoms are bloating, diarrhea, gas, nausea and abdominal cramps. Unfortunately, the recommended treatment is a lactose-free diet. If you avoid all dairy products you should also take calcium supplements. You can also buy lactase drops or tablets which can sometimes help you digest dairy products, if taken before eating them. If you're lactose intolerant, you'll likely find yogurt much more digestible than milk. That's because those friendly bacteria digest some of the milk sugar in yogurt, so there's less left to irritate you. There are also a range of lactose-free dairy products, like Lactaid milk, and soy-based products that you can substitute in. You shouldn't have any trouble following the 17 Day Diet with this food sensitivity.

Q. I have to be on a gluten-free diet. What are some foods that are naturally gluten-free?

A. For background, about 1 out of 133 people in the United States has celiac disease, an autoimmune intestinal disorder that causes severe allergies to proteins found in wheat and related grains. Even more people are gluten intolerant. For people with severe allergies to gluten, it's the difference between life and death, and a gluten-free diet is the only treatment. It prevents the complications of untreated celiac disease, such as osteoporosis, anemia, certain forms of cancer and even death. For people with intolerances to gluten, the benefits of a gluten-free diet are many: fewer sinus infections, more energy, less brain fog or less gastrointestinal upset. Some people lose weight on a gluten-free diet, but that may be because many high-calorie foods contain wheat, which is a carbohydrate.

Here is a partial list of gluten-free foods:

- Milk (nonfat dry milk)
- 100 percent vegetable juices
- Fresh fruits and vegetables that are not coated with a wax or resin that contains gluten
- A variety of single-ingredient foods: eggs, lentils, seeds like flax, tree nuts like almonds, gluten-free grains like corn, meats, fresh fish and fresh shellfish
- Gluten-free prepared foods such as bread, pastas, and special cereals

Foods that are not gluten-free include:

- Barley, common wheat, rye, spelt, kamut, triticale
- Farina, vital gluten, semolina, malt vinegar

As for oatmeal, no one agrees yet whether people with celiac disease can eat it or not. Research data suggests that the majority of people with celiac disease can tolerate a daily intake of a limited amount (e.g., 50 grams) of oats that are free of gluten from wheat, rye, barley or their crossbred hybrids.

By the way, if you're on a gluten-free diet, you can easily follow the 17 Day Diet by making food substitutions to include gluten-free products.

Keep those cards and letters coming . . . and visit me on the 17 Day website, www.the17daydiet.com, for more help and advice on how to live the diet and stay healthy and fit.

Appendix:

THE 17 DAY DIET JOURNAL

Use this special set of journal pages to write your own 17 Day Diet success story!

Tracking your diet is one of the best ways I know to help you achieve your weight-loss goals. In one study from the *American Journal of Preventive Medicine*, dieters who regularly recorded what they ate and when they exercised lost nearly twice as much weight as those who didn't keep track. I think there are a couple of different reasons for this: The first one is that recording how many doughnuts or bags of chips you've snacked on over the course of a week can be a real eye-opener. When your eating habits are staring at you from the page, it's hard to deny that the calories of sweets and fried foods all add up. Keeping a journal also makes it harder to cheat. Sure, you can lie when you fill out your journal, but YOU still know the truth, and for a lot of people, that's motivation enough to stay honest.

But the 17 Day Diet Journal isn't meant to be your police scanner—"We've got Twinkies on 2nd Avenue; send backup"—it's supposed to be your tool for success. Because the 17 Day Diet relies on body confusion to keep your metabolism guessing, your diet will vary from day to day. Using a journal can help you make sure you are getting the gist of low-calorie and high-calorie days, and if you are following my sample meal plans, this journal gives you a place to write it all down and add your own adjustments and notes. Plus you can use the hunger ratings column to be sure that you are truly hungry when you're eating, and that you aren't too full when you're done. Just circle the number that best fits your hunger or fullness level. For Dr. Mike's Hunger/Fullness Meter, see page 44.

To help you get started, I have given you 17 days' worth of journal pages where you can record your progress on the Accelerate Cycle. Then, after that set, I've included one more blank set that you can photocopy and fill out as many times as you want to track your progress through the other cycles.

Your Servings-Per-Day Cheat Sheet

	CYCLE 1: ACCELERATE	CYCLE 2: ACTIVATE	CYCLE 3: ACHIEVE	CYCLE 4: ARRIVE
Lean Proteins	Eat as much as you want	Eat as much as you want	Eat as much as you want	Enjoy the meal plans from Cycles 1 to 3 during the week. On weekends, employ strategic cheating!
Cleansing Vegetables	Eat as much as you want	Eat as much as you want	Eat as much as you want	
Low-Sugar Fruits	2 servings/ day	2 servings/ day	2 servings/ day	
Probiotic Foods	2 servings/ day	2 servings/ day	2 servings/ day	
Friendly Fats	1 to 2 tablespoons/ day	1 to 2 tablespoons/ day	1 to 2 tablespoons/ day	
Natural Starches	None (yet!)	2 servings/ day*	2 servings/ day	
Alcohol	None	None	Drink sparingly	Up to 1 or 2 drinks daily on weekends

*Only on Activate days, which alternate with Accelerate days on Cycle 2.

Accelerate Cycle, Day 1

Food Log

DATE: _____

	FOODS/DRINKS	TIME	HUNGER BEFORE	HUNGER AFTER
Breakfast			① ② ③ ④	① ② ③ ④
	NOTES:			
Lunch			① ② ③ ④	① ② ③ ④
	NOTES:			
Dinner			① ② ③ ④	① ② ③ ④
	NOTES:			
Snacks			① ② ③ ④	① ② ③ ④
	NOTES:			

Water Meter

Check a box for each 8-ounce glass you drink today.

☐ ☐ ☐ ☐ ☐ ☐ ☐ ☐

Exercise Log

Exercise (aerobic, strength, yoga, etc.)	Time/Duration	Weights Used/Other Notes

Additional Notes

Record your blood sugar, track your medications or make other notes here.

_____

_____

_____

_____

_____

_____

_____

Accelerate Cycle, Day 2

Food Log

DATE: _____

	FOODS/DRINKS	TIME	HUNGER BEFORE	HUNGER AFTER
Breakfast			① ② ③ ④	① ② ③ ④
	NOTES:			
Lunch			① ② ③ ④	① ② ③ ④
	NOTES:			
Dinner			① ② ③ ④	① ② ③ ④
	NOTES:			
Snacks			① ② ③ ④	① ② ③ ④
	NOTES:			

Water Meter

Check a box for each 8-ounce glass you drink today.

☐ ☐ ☐ ☐ ☐ ☐ ☐ ☐

Exercise Log

Exercise (aerobic, strength, yoga, etc.)	Time/Duration	Weights Used/Other Notes

Additional Notes

Record your blood sugar, track your medications or make other notes here.

Accelerate Cycle, Day 3

Food Log

DATE:_____

	FOODS/DRINKS	TIME	HUNGER BEFORE	HUNGER AFTER
Breakfast			① ② ③ ④	① ② ③ ④
	NOTES:			
Lunch			① ② ③ ④	① ② ③ ④
	NOTES:			
Dinner			① ② ③ ④	① ② ③ ④
	NOTES:			
Snacks			① ② ③ ④	① ② ③ ④
	NOTES:			

Water Meter

Check a box for each 8-ounce glass you drink today.

☐ ☐ ☐ ☐ ☐ ☐ ☐ ☐

Exercise Log

Exercise (aerobic, strength, yoga, etc.)	Time/Duration	Weights Used/Other Notes

Additional Notes

Record your blood sugar, track your medications or make other notes here.

_____

_____

_____

_____

_____

_____

_____

Accelerate Cycle, Day 4

Food Log

DATE:_____

	FOODS/DRINKS	TIME	HUNGER BEFORE	HUNGER AFTER
Breakfast			① ② ③ ④	① ② ③ ④
	NOTES:			
Lunch			① ② ③ ④	① ② ③ ④
	NOTES:			
Dinner			① ② ③ ④	① ② ③ ④
	NOTES:			
Snacks			① ② ③ ④	① ② ③ ④
	NOTES:			

Water Meter

Check a box for each 8-ounce glass you drink today.

Exercise Log

Exercise (aerobic, strength, yoga, etc.)	Time/Duration	Weights Used/Other Notes

Additional Notes

Record your blood sugar, track your medications or make other notes here.

Accelerate Cycle, Day 5

Food Log

DATE:_____

	FOODS/DRINKS	TIME	HUNGER BEFORE	HUNGER AFTER
Breakfast			① ② ③ ④	① ② ③ ④
	NOTES:			
Lunch			① ② ③ ④	① ② ③ ④
	NOTES:			
Dinner			① ② ③ ④	① ② ③ ④
	NOTES:			
Snacks			① ② ③ ④	① ② ③ ④
	NOTES:			

Water Meter

Check a box for each 8-ounce glass you drink today.

☐ ☐ ☐ ☐ ☐ ☐ ☐ ☐

Exercise Log

Exercise (aerobic, strength, yoga, etc.)	Time/Duration	Weights Used/Other Notes

Additional Notes

Record your blood sugar, track your medications or make other notes here.

Accelerate Cycle, Day 6

Food Log

DATE:_____

	FOODS/DRINKS	TIME	HUNGER BEFORE	HUNGER AFTER
Breakfast			① ② ③ ④	① ② ③ ④
	NOTES:			
Lunch			① ② ③ ④	① ② ③ ④
	NOTES:			
Dinner			① ② ③ ④	① ② ③ ④
	NOTES:			
Snacks			① ② ③ ④	① ② ③ ④
	NOTES:			

Water Meter

Check a box for each 8-ounce glass you drink today.

Exercise Log

Exercise (aerobic, strength, yoga, etc.)	Time/Duration	Weights Used/Other Notes

Additional Notes

Record your blood sugar, track your medications or make other notes here.

_____

_____

_____

_____

_____

_____

_____

Accelerate Cycle, Day 7

Food Log

DATE:_____

	FOODS/DRINKS	TIME	HUNGER BEFORE	HUNGER AFTER
Breakfast			① ② ③ ④	① ② ③ ④
	NOTES:			
Lunch			① ② ③ ④	① ② ③ ④
	NOTES:			
Dinner			① ② ③ ④	① ② ③ ④
	NOTES:			
Snacks			① ② ③ ④	① ② ③ ④
	NOTES:			

Water Meter

Check a box for each 8-ounce glass you drink today.

☐ ☐ ☐ ☐ ☐ ☐ ☐ ☐ ☐

Exercise Log

Exercise (aerobic, strength, yoga, etc.)	Time/Duration	Weights Used/Other Notes

Additional Notes

Record your blood sugar, track your medications or make other notes here.

Accelerate Cycle, Day 8

Food Log

DATE:_____

	FOODS/DRINKS	TIME	HUNGER BEFORE	HUNGER AFTER
Breakfast			① ② ③ ④	① ② ③ ④
	NOTES:			
Lunch			① ② ③ ④	① ② ③ ④
	NOTES:			
Dinner			① ② ③ ④	① ② ③ ④
	NOTES:			
Snacks			① ② ③ ④	① ② ③ ④
	NOTES:			

Water Meter

Check a box for each 8-ounce glass you drink today.

☐ ☐ ☐ ☐ ☐ ☐ ☐ ☐

Exercise Log

Exercise (aerobic, strength, yoga, etc.)	Time/Duration	Weights Used/Other Notes

Additional Notes

Record your blood sugar, track your medications or make other notes here.

_____

_____

_____

_____

_____

_____

Accelerate Cycle, Day 9

Food Log

DATE:_____

	FOODS/DRINKS	TIME	HUNGER BEFORE	HUNGER AFTER
Breakfast			① ② ③ ④	① ② ③ ④
	NOTES:			
Lunch			① ② ③ ④	① ② ③ ④
	NOTES:			
Dinner			① ② ③ ④	① ② ③ ④
	NOTES:			
Snacks			① ② ③ ④	① ② ③ ④
	NOTES:			

Water Meter

Check a box for each 8-ounce glass you drink today.

☐　☐　☐　☐　☐　☐　☐　☐

Exercise Log

Exercise (aerobic, strength, yoga, etc.)	Time/Duration	Weights Used/Other Notes

Additional Notes

Record your blood sugar, track your medications or make other notes here.

_____

_____

_____

_____

_____

_____

_____

Accelerate Cycle, Day 10

Food Log

DATE:_____

	FOODS/DRINKS	TIME	HUNGER BEFORE	HUNGER AFTER
Breakfast			① ② ③ ④	① ② ③ ④
	NOTES:			
Lunch			① ② ③ ④	① ② ③ ④
	NOTES:			
Dinner			① ② ③ ④	① ② ③ ④
	NOTES:			
Snacks			① ② ③ ④	① ② ③ ④
	NOTES:			

Water Meter

Check a box for each 8-ounce glass you drink today.

☐ ☐ ☐ ☐ ☐ ☐ ☐ ☐

Exercise Log

Exercise (aerobic, strength, yoga, etc.)	Time/Duration	Weights Used/Other Notes

Additional Notes

Record your blood sugar, track your medications or make other notes here.

_____

_____

_____

_____

_____

_____

_____

Accelerate Cycle, Day 11

Food Log

DATE:_____

	FOODS/DRINKS	TIME	HUNGER BEFORE	HUNGER AFTER
Breakfast			① ② ③ ④	① ② ③ ④
	NOTES:			
Lunch			① ② ③ ④	① ② ③ ④
	NOTES:			
Dinner			① ② ③ ④	① ② ③ ④
	NOTES:			
Snacks			① ② ③ ④	① ② ③ ④
	NOTES:			

Water Meter

Check a box for each 8-ounce glass you drink today.

Exercise Log

Exercise (aerobic, strength, yoga, etc.)	Time/Duration	Weights Used/Other Notes

Additional Notes

Record your blood sugar, track your medications or make other notes here.

_____

_____

_____

_____

_____

_____

_____

Accelerate Cycle, Day 12

Food Log

DATE:_____

	FOODS/DRINKS	TIME	HUNGER BEFORE	HUNGER AFTER
Breakfast			① ② ③ ④	① ② ③ ④
	NOTES:			
Lunch			① ② ③ ④	① ② ③ ④
	NOTES:			
Dinner			① ② ③ ④	① ② ③ ④
	NOTES:			
Snacks			① ② ③ ④	① ② ③ ④
	NOTES:			

Water Meter

Check a box for each 8-ounce glass you drink today.

☐ ☐ ☐ ☐ ☐ ☐ ☐ ☐

Exercise Log

Exercise (aerobic, strength, yoga, etc.)	Time/Duration	Weights Used/Other Notes

Additional Notes

Record your blood sugar, track your medications or make other notes here.

_____

_____

_____

_____

_____

_____

_____

Accelerate Cycle, Day 13

Food Log

DATE:_____

	FOODS/DRINKS	TIME	HUNGER BEFORE	HUNGER AFTER
Breakfast			① ② ③ ④	① ② ③ ④
	NOTES:			
Lunch			① ② ③ ④	① ② ③ ④
	NOTES:			
Dinner			① ② ③ ④	① ② ③ ④
	NOTES:			
Snacks			① ② ③ ④	① ② ③ ④
	NOTES:			

Water Meter

Check a box for each 8-ounce glass you drink today.

☐ ☐ ☐ ☐ ☐ ☐ ☐ ☐

Exercise Log

Exercise (aerobic, strength, yoga, etc.)	Time/Duration	Weights Used/Other Notes

Additional Notes

Record your blood sugar, track your medications or make other notes here.

_____

_____

_____

_____

_____

_____

Accelerate Cycle, Day 14

Food Log

DATE:_____

	FOODS/DRINKS	TIME	HUNGER BEFORE	HUNGER AFTER
Breakfast			① ② ③ ④	① ② ③ ④
	NOTES:			
Lunch			① ② ③ ④	① ② ③ ④
	NOTES:			
Dinner			① ② ③ ④	① ② ③ ④
	NOTES:			
Snacks			① ② ③ ④	① ② ③ ④
	NOTES:			

Water Meter

Check a box for each 8-ounce glass you drink today.

☐ ☐ ☐ ☐ ☐ ☐ ☐ ☐

Exercise Log

Exercise (aerobic, strength, yoga, etc.)	Time/Duration	Weights Used/Other Notes

Additional Notes

Record your blood sugar, track your medications or make other notes here.

Accelerate Cycle, Day 15

Food Log

DATE:_____

	FOODS/DRINKS	TIME	HUNGER BEFORE	HUNGER AFTER
Breakfast			① ② ③ ④	① ② ③ ④
	NOTES:			
Lunch			① ② ③ ④	① ② ③ ④
	NOTES:			
Dinner			① ② ③ ④	① ② ③ ④
	NOTES:			
Snacks			① ② ③ ④	① ② ③ ④
	NOTES:			

Water Meter

Check a box for each 8-ounce glass you drink today.

☐ ☐ ☐ ☐ ☐ ☐ ☐ ☐

Exercise Log

Exercise (aerobic, strength, yoga, etc.)	Time/Duration	Weights Used/Other Notes

Additional Notes

Record your blood sugar, track your medications or make other notes here.

Accelerate Cycle, Day 16

Food Log

DATE:_____

	FOODS/DRINKS	TIME	HUNGER BEFORE	HUNGER AFTER
Breakfast			① ② ③ ④	① ② ③ ④
	NOTES:			
Lunch			① ② ③ ④	① ② ③ ④
	NOTES:			
Dinner			① ② ③ ④	① ② ③ ④
	NOTES:			
Snacks			① ② ③ ④	① ② ③ ④
	NOTES:			

Water Meter

Check a box for each 8-ounce glass you drink today.

☐ ☐ ☐ ☐ ☐ ☐ ☐ ☐

Exercise Log

Exercise (aerobic, strength, yoga, etc.)	Time/Duration	Weights Used/Other Notes

Additional Notes

Record your blood sugar, track your medications or make other notes here.

Accelerate Cycle, Day 17

Food Log

DATE:_____

	FOODS/DRINKS	TIME	HUNGER BEFORE	HUNGER AFTER
Breakfast			① ② ③ ④	① ② ③ ④
	NOTES:			
Lunch			① ② ③ ④	① ② ③ ④
	NOTES:			
Dinner			① ② ③ ④	① ② ③ ④
	NOTES:			
Snacks			① ② ③ ④	① ② ③ ④
	NOTES:			

Water Meter

Check a box for each 8-ounce glass you drink today.

☐ ☐ ☐ ☐ ☐ ☐ ☐ ☐

Exercise Log

Exercise (aerobic, strength, yoga, etc.)	Time/Duration	Weights Used/Other Notes

Additional Notes

Record your blood sugar, track your medications or make other notes here.

_____

_____

_____

_____

_____

_____

_____

Cycle_____ Day_____

Food Log

DATE:_____

	FOODS/DRINKS	TIME	HUNGER BEFORE	HUNGER AFTER
Breakfast			① ② ③ ④	① ② ③ ④
	NOTES:			
Lunch			① ② ③ ④	① ② ③ ④
	NOTES:			
Dinner			① ② ③ ④	① ② ③ ④
	NOTES:			
Snacks			① ② ③ ④	① ② ③ ④
	NOTES:			

Water Meter

Check a box for each 8-ounce glass you drink today.

☐ ☐ ☐ ☐ ☐ ☐ ☐ ☐

Exercise Log

Exercise (aerobic, strength, yoga, etc.)	Time/Duration	Weights Used/Other Notes

Additional Notes

Record your blood sugar, track your medications or make other notes here.

Resources

Much of the material in this book comes from computer searches of medical databases of abstracts, medical news reports in both popular and specialized publications, as well as published scientific reports in peer-reviewed journals.

Chapter 1: Just Give Me 17 Days

Binks, M. 2005. Duke study reports sex, self-esteem diminish for morbidly obese. *CDS Review* 98(4):28–29.

Bui, C., 2010. Acute effect of a single high-fat meal on forearm blood flow, blood pressure and heart rate in healthy male Asians and Caucasians: a pilot study. *The Southeast Asia Journal of Tropical Health and Public Health* 41:490–500.

Claessens, M., et al. 2009. The effect of a low-fat, high-protein or high-carbohydrate ad libitum diet on weight loss maintenance and metabolic risk factors. *International Journal of Obesity* 33:296–304.

Gunn, D. A. 2009. Why some women look young for their age. *PLoS One* 4:e8021.

Hanninen, O., et al. 1992. Effects of eating an uncooked vegetable diet for one week. *Appetite* 19:243–254.

Henkin, Y., and Shai, I. 2003. Dietary treatment of hypercholesterolemia: can we predict long-term success? *Journal of the American College of Nutrition* 22:555–561.

Janiszewski, P. M., and Ross, R. 2010. Effects of weight loss among metabolically healthy obese men and women. *Diabetes Care* 33:1957–1959.

Jenkins, D. J., et al. 2009. The effect of a plant-based low-carbohydrate ("Eco-Atkins") diet on body weight and blood lipid concentrations in hyperlipidemic subjects. *Archives of Internal Medicine* 169:1046–1054.

Johnston, C.S., 2002. Postprandial thermogenesis is increased 100% on a high-protein, low-fat diet versus a high-carbohydrate, low-fat diet in healthy, young women. *Journal of the American College of Nutrition* 21:55–61.

Kiortsis, D. N., et al. 2001. Changes in lipoprotein(a) levels and hormonal correlations during a weight reduction program. *Nutrition, Metabolism, and Cardiovascular Diseases* 11:153–157.

Laaksonen, D. E., et al. 2003. Relationships between changes in abdominal fat distribution and insulin sensitivity during a very low calorie diet in abdominally obese men and women. *Nutrition, Metabolism, and Cardiovascular Diseases* 13:349–356.

Lapidus, L. 1984. Distribution of adipose tissue and risk of cardiovascular disease and death: a 12-year follow up of participants in the population study of women in Gothenburg, Sweden. *British Medical Journal* 289:1257.

Leigh, Gibson E., and Green, M. W. 2002. Nutritional influences on cognitive function: mechanisms of susceptibility. *Nutrition Research Reviews* 15:169–206.

Maconochie, N. 2007. Risk factors for first trimester miscarriage—results from a UK-population-based case-control study. *BJOG* 114:170–186.

Nackers, L. M., et al. 2010. The association between rate of initial weight loss and long-term success in obesity treatment: does slow and steady win the race? *International Journal of Behavioral Medicine* 17:161–167.

Nowson, C. A., 2003. Dietary approaches to reduce blood pressure in a community setting: a randomised crossover study. *Asia Pacific Journal of Clinical Nutrition* 12 Suppl:S19.

Rudkowska, I., et al. 2008. Cholesterol-lowering efficacy of plant sterols in low-fat yogurt consumed as a snack or with a meal. *Journal of the American College of Nutrition* 27:588–595.

Sheets, V., and Ajmere, K. 2005. Are romantic partners a source of college students' weight concern? *Eating Behaviors* 6:1–9.

Tran, T. T. 2008. Beneficial effects of subcutaneous fat transplantation on metabolism. *Cell Metabolism* 7:410–420.

Chapter 2: Burn, Baby, Burn

Diamant, M., 2010. Do nutrient-gut-microbiota interactions play a role in human obesity, insulin resistance and type 2 diabetes? *Obesity Review,* August 13.

Kim, D. H., et al. 2010. Peptide designed to elicit apoptosis in adipose tissue endothelium reduces food intake and body weight. *Diabetes* 59:907–915.

McCrory, M. A., et al. 1999. Dietary variety within food groups: association with energy intake and body fatness in men and women. *American Journal of Clinical Nutrition* 69:440–447.

Pataky, Z. 2009. Gut microbiota, responsible for our body weight? *Revue Medicale Suisse* 5:662–664, 666.

Scarpellini, E. 2010. Gut microbiota and obesity. *Internal and Emergency Medicine* 5 Suppl 1:S53–56.

Yang, C. S., and Wang, X. 2010. Green tea and cancer prevention. *Nutrition and Cancer* 62(7):931–937.

Chapter 3: Cycle 1: Accelerate

Tremblay, A., et al. 2004. Thermogenesis and weight loss in obese individuals: a primary association with organochlorine pollution. *International Journal of Obesity and Related Metabolic Disorders* 28(7):936–939.

Chapter 4: Cycle 2: Activate

Jakulj, F. 2007. A high-fat meal increases cardiovascular reactivity to psychological stress in healthy young adults. *Journal of Nutrition* 137:935–939.

Liu, H. 2010. Fructose induces transketolase flux to promote pancreatic cancer growth. *Cancer Research* 70:6368–6376.

Varady, K. A. 2007. Alternate-day fasting and chronic disease prevention: a review of human and animal trials. *American Journal of Clinical Nutrition* 86:7–13.

Westerterp-Planteng, M. S., et al. 2005. Sensory and gastrointestinal satiety effects of capsaicin on food intake. *International Journal of Obesity* 29:682–688.

Chapter 5: Cycle 3: Achieve

Di Blasio, A. 2010. Effects of the time of day of walking on dietary behaviour, body composition and aerobic fitness in post-menopausal women. *The Journal of Sports Medicine and Physical Fitness* 50:196–201.

Fischer-Posovszky, P. 2010. Resveratrol regulates human adipocyte number and function in a Sirt1-dependent manner. *American Journal of Clinical Nutrition* 92:5–15.

Fuchs, N. K. 2002. Liposuction lowers cholesterol. *Women's Health Letter.* Soundview Publications.

Kristal, A. R. 2005. Yoga practice is associated with attenuated weight gain in healthy, middle-aged men and women. *Alternative Therapies in Health and Medicine* 11:28–33.

National Weight Control Registry. www.nwcr.ws/Research/default.htm.

Rolls, B. J., et al. 2004. Salad and satiety: energy density and portion size of a first-course salad affect energy intake at lunch. *Journal of the American Dietetic Association* 104:1570–1576.

Vgontzas, A.N. 2007. Daytime napping after a night of sleep loss decreases sleepiness, improves performance, and causes beneficial changes in cortisol and interleukin-6 secretion. *American Journal of Physiology, Endocrinology, and Metabolism* 292: E253–E261.

Chapter 8: The PMS Exception Diet

Benton, D., and Cook, R. 1991. The impact of selenium supplementation on mood. *Biological Psychiatry* 29:1092–1098.

Ghanbari, Z., et al. 2009. Effects of calcium supplement therapy in women with premenstrual syndrome. *Taiwan Journal Obstetrics and Gynecology* 48:124–129.

Hawkes, W. C., and Hornbostel, L. 1996. Effects of dietary selenium on mood in healthy men living in a metabolic research unit. *Biological Psychiatry* 39:121–128.

Hibbeln, J. R. 1998. Fish consumption and major depression. *The Lancet* 351:1213.

Hibbeln, J. R., and Salem, N. 1995. Dietary polyunsaturated fatty acids and depression: when cholesterol does not satisfy. *American Journal of Clinical Nutrition* 62:1–9.

Kalman, D., et al. 2009. A prospective, randomized, double-blind, placebo-controlled parallel-group dual site trial to evaluate the effects of a Bacillus coagulans-based product on functional intestinal gas symptoms. *BMC Gastroenterology* 18:85.

Chapter 10: Family Challenges

Morgan, D. V., et al. 1988. Mutual motivation. *Health*, August, 32–36.

Paisley, J,, et al. 2008. Dietary change: what are the responses and roles of significant others? *Journal of Nutrition Education and Behavior* 40:80–88.

Wallace, J. P. 1995. Twelve month adherence of adults who joined a fitness program with a spouse vs. without a spouse. *Journal of Sports Medicine and Physical Fitness* 35:206–213.

Chapter 11: Surviving Holidays

Andersson, I., et al. 1992. The Christmas factor in obesity therapy. *International Journal of Obesity and Related Metabolic Disorders* 16:013–1015.

Baker, R. C., et al. Weight control during the holidays: Highly consistent self-monitoring as a potentially useful coping mechanism. *Health Psychology* 17:367–370.

Chapter 13: Shift Work on the 17 Day Diet

Geliebter, A. 2000. Work-shift period and weight change. *Nutrition* 16:27–29.

Henderson, N. J., and Christopher D. B. B. 1998. An evaluation of the effectiveness of shift work preparation strategies. *New Zealand Journal of Psychology*. New Zealand Psychological Society.

Thorpy, M. J. 2010. Managing the patient with shift-work disorder. *The Journal of Family Practice* 59(1 Suppl):S24–31.

Chapter 15: Mister MD, Can You Please Tell Me More?

Checkoway, H., et al. 2002. Parkinson's disease risks associated with cigarette smoking, alcohol consumption, and caffeine intake. *American Journal of Epidemiology*. 155:732–738.

Marian, T., et al. 2000. Effect of dietary protein on bone loss in elderly men and women: The Framingham Osteoporosis Study. *Journal of Bone and Mineral Research* 15:2504–2512.

Shape Magazine. April 2009. Trying to quit smoking? Get moving.

Shengxu, L., et al. 2010. Physical activity attenuates the genetic predisposition to obesity in 20,000 men and women from EPIC-Norfolk prospective population study. *PloS Medicine* e1000332. doi:10.1371/journal.pmed.1000332.

van Dam, R. M., et al. 2006. Coffee, caffeine, and risk of type 2 diabetes: a prospective cohort study in younger and middle-aged U.S. women. *Diabetes Care* 29:398–403.

About the Author

Dr. Michael Rafael Moreno, better known as Dr. Mike, is a graduate of the University of California at Irvine and Hahnemann Medical School (now Drexel University). Following his residency at Kaiser Permanente in Fontana, California, Dr. Mike moved to San Diego, where he now practices family medicine and sits on the board of the San Diego Chapter of the American Academy of Family Physicians.

In 2008, Dr. Mike launched "Walk with Your Doc," which he participates in every Tuesday and Thursday morning before his workday begins. The program began when Dr. Mike offered to walk with a patient to motivate her to exercise, and has since grown into a thriving community.

Dr. Mike takes pride in being viewed not only as a doctor, but also as a friend and confidant.

"We've all pledged, promised and bullied ourselves to eat better and exercise more, but so many times even the best intentions fall short," Dr. Mike says. "I incorporate healthy habits into my work and home life, and you can too."

Index

. . . .

Underscored page references indicate boxed text.